Josef Johann Gross

Metabolic priority of milk production

Josef Johann Gross

Metabolic priority of milk production

Adaptation to lactational and nutrition induced negative energy balance in dairy cows

Südwestdeutscher Verlag für Hochschulschriften

Impressum/Imprint (nur für Deutschland/only for Germany)
Bibliografische Information der Deutschen Nationalbibliothek: Die Deutsche Nationalbibliothek verzeichnet diese Publikation in der Deutschen Nationalbibliografie; detaillierte bibliografische Daten sind im Internet über http://dnb.d-nb.de abrufbar.

Alle in diesem Buch genannten Marken und Produktnamen unterliegen warenzeichen-, marken- oder patentrechtlichem Schutz bzw. sind Warenzeichen oder eingetragene Warenzeichen der jeweiligen Inhaber. Die Wiedergabe von Marken, Produktnamen, Gebrauchsnamen, Handelsnamen, Warenbezeichnungen u.s.w. in diesem Werk berechtigt auch ohne besondere Kennzeichnung nicht zu der Annahme, dass solche Namen im Sinne der Warenzeichen- und Markenschutzgesetzgebung als frei zu betrachten wären und daher von jedermann benutzt werden dürften.

Coverbild: www.ingimage.com

Verlag: Südwestdeutscher Verlag für Hochschulschriften GmbH & Co. KG
Heinrich-Böcking-Str. 6-8, 66121 Saarbrücken, Deutschland
Telefon +49 681 37 20 271-1, Telefax +49 681 37 20 271-0
Email: info@svh-verlag.de

Approved by: München, TU, Diss., 2011

Herstellung in Deutschland:
Schaltungsdienst Lange o.H.G., Berlin
Books on Demand GmbH, Norderstedt
Reha GmbH, Saarbrücken
Amazon Distribution GmbH, Leipzig
ISBN: 978-3-8381-3139-9

Imprint (only for USA, GB)
Bibliographic information published by the Deutsche Nationalbibliothek: The Deutsche Nationalbibliothek lists this publication in the Deutsche Nationalbibliografie; detailed bibliographic data are available in the Internet at http://dnb.d-nb.de.

Any brand names and product names mentioned in this book are subject to trademark, brand or patent protection and are trademarks or registered trademarks of their respective holders. The use of brand names, product names, common names, trade names, product descriptions etc. even without a particular marking in this works is in no way to be construed to mean that such names may be regarded as unrestricted in respect of trademark and brand protection legislation and could thus be used by anyone.

Cover image: www.ingimage.com

Publisher: Südwestdeutscher Verlag für Hochschulschriften GmbH & Co. KG
Heinrich-Böcking-Str. 6-8, 66121 Saarbrücken, Germany
Phone +49 681 37 20 271-1, Fax +49 681 37 20 271-0
Email: info@svh-verlag.de

Printed in the U.S.A.
Printed in the U.K. by (see last page)
ISBN: 978-3-8381-3139-9

Copyright © 2012 by the author and Südwestdeutscher Verlag für Hochschulschriften GmbH & Co. KG and licensors
All rights reserved. Saarbrücken 2012

Table of contents

Table of contents I
List of tables II
List of figures III
Abbreviations V
Abstract VII
Zusammenfassung XI
1. Introduction 1
2. Material and Methods 3
    2.1   Experimental design, animals and housing 3
    2.2   Feeding regimen 4
    2.3   Analysis of feed samples and determination of energy and protein balance 6
    2.4   Milk samples and analysis 8
    2.5   Body weight and body condition parameters 9
    2.6   Animal health 9
    2.7   Blood samples and analysis 9
    2.8   Liver samples and analysis 10
    2.9   Statistical evaluation 11
        2.9.1 Performance, metabolic and health status data 12
        2.9.2 Hormones and gene expression data 12
        2.9.3 Milk FA and their relation to energy status 13
3. Results and Discussion 15
    3.1   Adaptation of performance parameters to a NEB 15
    3.2   Adaptation of metabolites to a NEB 28
    3.3   Adaptations of endocrine and hepatic gene expression parameters to a NEB 32
    3.4   Milk fatty acids and their relation to energy status 46
4. Conclusions 59
5. References 61
6. Acknowledgements 71
7. Overview scientific communications 73
8. Appendix 75

List of tables

Table 1. Composition of the experimental diets and the concentrate 4

Table 2. Nutrient values of experimental diets and concentrate 5

Table 3. Nutrient value of forages used in the experimental diets and the concentrate 6

Table 4. Fatty acid composition of the experimental diets and the concentrate 7

Table 5. PCR primer information, annealing temperature, and the PCR product length for genes analyzed in liver samples 11

Table 6. Occurrence (quantity) of health disorders during experimental periods 28

Table 7. Changes in milk fatty acid (FA) composition in week 1, 4, 6, 12 (all animals), 17 and 21 (control group) post partum 47

Table 8. Changes in milk fatty acid (FA) composition for feed-restricted and control cows during feed-restriction and realimentation 52

Table 9. Direction of adaptation of endocrine factors and liver gene expression parameters during the two stages of a NEB 60

List of figures

Figure 1. Experimental design and sampling schedule 3
Figure 2. Dry matter intake (DMI; kg/d) in cows during the experimental periods 15
Figure 3. Energy intake (MJ NEL/d) in cows during the experimental periods 16
Figure 4. Milk yield (kg/d) in cows during the experimental periods 17
Figure 5. Energy balance (EB; MJ NEL/d) in cows during the experimental periods 17
Figure 6. Available crude protein balance (ACP; g/d) in cows during the
 experimental periods 19
Figure 7. Milk fat and protein content (%) in cows during the experimental periods 20
Figure 8. Milk fat yield (g/d) in cows during the experimental periods 21
Figure 9. Milk protein yield (g/d) in cows during the experimental periods 22
Figure 10. Milk fat-protein ratio in cows during the experimental periods 22
Figure 11. Milk lactose content (%) in cows during the experimental periods......................... 23
Figure 12. Body weight (BW; kg) of cows during the experimental periods 24
Figure 13. Body condition score (BCS) of cows during the experimental periods 25
Figure 14. Backfat thickness (BFT; mm) of cows during the experimental periods 26
Figure 15. Muscle diameter (MD; mm) of the longissimus dorsi muscle in cows
 during the experimental periods 27
Figure 16. Plasma glucose concentration (mmol/L) in cows during the
 experimental periods 29
Figure 17. Plasma NEFA concentration (mmol/L) in cows during the
 experimental periods 30
Figure 18. Plasma BHBA concentration (mmol/L) in cows during the
 experimental periods 31
Figure 19. Plasma concentration of insulin (μU/mL) in cows during the
 experimental periods 32
Figure 20. Relative liver mRNA abundance (delta CT, $\log_2$) of insulin receptor (INSR)
 in cows over the time points 33
Figure 21. The revised quantitative insulin sensitivity check index (RQUICKI) in
 cows during the experimental periods 34
Figure 22. Plasma concentration of growth hormone (GH; μg/L) in cows during the
 experimental periods 36
Figure 23. Relative liver mRNA abundance (delta CT, $\log_2$) of GH receptor 1A
 (GHR 1A) in cows over the time points 37

List of figures

Figure 24. Plasma concentration of insulin-like growth factor-I (IGF-I; ng/mL) in cows during the experimental periods 38

Figure 25. Relative liver mRNA abundance (delta CT, $\log_2$) of IGF-I in cows over the time points 38

Figure 26. Relative liver mRNA abundance (delta CT, $\log_2$) of IGF-I receptor (IGF-IR) in cows over the time points 39

Figure 27. Relative liver mRNA abundance (delta CT, $\log_2$) of IGF binding protein-1 (IGFBP-1) in cows over the time points 40

Figure 28. Relative liver mRNA abundance (delta CT, $\log_2$) of IGFBP-2 in cows over the time points 41

Figure 29. Relative liver mRNA abundance (delta CT, $\log_2$) of IGFBP-3 in cows over the time points 42

Figure 30. Plasma concentration of leptin (ng/mL) in cows during the experimental periods 43

Figure 31. Plasma concentration of 3,5,3'-trijodthyronine (T_3; nmol/L) in cows during the experimental periods 44

Figure 32. Plasma concentration of thyroxine (T_4; nmol/L) in cows during the experimental periods 45

Figure 33. Ratio of T_3:T_4 in cows during the experimental periods 46

Figure 34. Changes in saturated FA, monounsaturated FA and polyunsaturated FA in milk fat during the first 21 weeks of lactation in dairy cows 49

Figure 35. Changes in saturated FA, monounsaturated FA and polyunsaturated FA in milk fat of feed-restricted and control cows during feed-restriction (week 15 to 17 post partum) and subsequent realimentation (week 18 to 19 post partum) 51

Abbreviations

acetyl-CoA	acetyl-coenzyme A
ACP	available crude protein
ADF	acid detergent fiber
ADL	lignin
a.m.	morning
a.p.	ante partum
ATP	adenosine triphosphate
AUC	area under the curve
BCS	body condition score
BFT	backfat thickness
BHBA	beta-hydroxybutyrate
BW	body weight
C	control
cDNA	copy deoxyribonucleic acid
CLA	conjugated linoleic acid
c	centi
CONC	concentrate
CP	crude protein
CT	threshold cycle
d	day
°C	degree Celsius
Δ	delta
DIM	days in milk
DLG	German agricultural society
DM	dry matter
DMI	dry matter intake
EB	energy balance
e.g.	for example
FA	fatty acid
$FADH_2$	reduced flavin adenine dinucleotide
FAME	fatty acid methyl ester
FAO	Food and Agriculture Organization of the United Nations
FM	fresh matter
g	gram
G	gauge
GAPDH	glyceraldehyde-3-phosphate dehydrogenase
GfE	German Society of Nutrition Physiology
GH	growth hormone
GHR 1A	growth hormone receptor 1A
GLUT	glucose transporter
h	hour
i.e.	id est, that is
IGF-I	insulin-like growth factor-I
IGF-IR	insulin-like growth factor-I receptor
IGFBP	insulin-like growth factor binding protein
INSR	insulin receptor
k	kilo
K_3EDTA	tripotassium-ethylene-diamine-tetra-acetate
L	liter

log	logarithm
m	milli/meter
MD	diameter of the longissimus dorsi muscle
MHz	megahertz
µ	micro
min	minute
MJ	megajoule
mRNA	messenger ribonucleic acid
MUFA	monounsaturated fatty acid
n	nano/number
NADH	reduced nicotinamide adenine dinucleotide
NDF	neutral detergent fiber
NEB	negative energy balance
NEFA	nonesterified fatty acid
NEL	net energy lactation
NFC	nonfiber carbohydrates
NRC	National Research Council
P	level of significance
%	percent
p	pico
PCR	polymerase chain reaction
p.m.	evening
PMR	partial mixed ration
p.p.	post partum
PUFA	polyunsaturated fatty acid
R	feed-restricted
RNA	ribonucleic acid
RNB	ruminal nitrogen balance
RQUICKI	revised quantitative insulin sensitivity check index
s	second
SD	standard deviation
SEM	standard error of the means
SFA	saturated fatty acid
T_3	3,5,3'-trijodthyronine
T_4	thyroxine
TMR	total mixed ration
U	unit
UBQ	ubiquitin
VLDL	very low density lipoprotein
vs.	versus

Abstract

Homeorhetic and homeostatic control in dairy cows are essential to adapt to alterations in physiological and environmental conditions. A negative energy balance (NEB) usually occurs in dairy cows after calving but can also appear later in lactation during periods of insufficient feed supply. Cows need to adapt to a NEB to maintain lactation and vital functions. The aim of the present study was to investigate the differential adaptation of performance, metabolism and endocrine systems to a lactational and a nutrition induced NEB of dairy cows.

Fifty multiparous Holstein cows (3.2 ± 1.4 lactations) were studied in three periods (period 1 = week 3 ante partum up to week 12 post partum; period 2 = feed-restriction for 3 weeks beginning at 98 ± 7 days in milk with a feed-restricted and control group with 25 cows each; and period 3 = subsequent realimentation period for the feed-restricted group for 8 weeks). Throughout the experiment all cows obtained a partial mixed ration (PMR; based on maize silage, grass silage, hay and concentrate) ad libitum, except for restricted cows during period 2. For period 2, the NEB was induced by individual limitation of feed quantity and reduction of dietary energy density. Additional concentrate was fed individually when milk yield was above 21 kg/d, except during the restriction period, where it was set by 0.4 kg/d. Feed intake and milk yield were recorded daily, body weight (BW) weekly. Blood samples were taken once a week, milk samples twice a week. Liver biopsies were taken in week 3 a.p., week 1 and 4 p.p. (period 1) and in week 0 and 3 of period 2. EB of each cow was calculated from daily feed intake, maintenance requirement and milk yield.

Feed intake, energy balance, milk yield and milk solubles

DMI increased steadily from 14.9 ± 0.2 kg/d (week 1 p.p.) to over 22 kg/d in weeks 7 to 12 of period 1. NEB was highest in week 1 p.p. with -46.1 MJ NEL/d and cows covered only 70% of their energetic requirements by feed intake. EB turned positive in week 9 p.p. over all cows and reached a level of 103% of the demand before experimental period 2. During period 2, restricted cows had a mean DMI of 10.3 kg/d and covered herefrom 51% of their energy requirements, whereas control cows had a DMI of 21.1 kg/d and an energy balance of 104%. In week 1 of realimentation (period 3), control cows still had a higher feed intake than restricted cows (20.4 vs. 18.7 kg/d; $P < 0.05$). EB for restricted cows turned positive again in week 2 of period 3 and averaged 109% of the calculated demand (control cows 108%) until the end of the study. Milk yield started at 27.5 ± 0.7 kg/d in week 1 p.p., peaked in week 6 p.p. (39.5 ± 0.8 kg/d) and decreased to 32.8 ± 0.8 kg/d in week 12 p.p.. During period 2, restricted cows had a only a slightly lower milk yield (27.4 kg/d) than control cows (30.5 kg/d; $P < 0.05$) despite the high nutrition induced NEB. Milk yield of restricted cows increased in the first week of period 3 and did not differ from the level of control cows. Milk fat percentage was highest in week 1 p.p. (5.48%) and dropped to 4.00% in week 7 p.p.. Within the first week of period 2, milk fat content rose from 4.30 to 4.63% ($P < 0.10$). However, there were no differences between the groups during the rest of period 2 and 3. Milk protein content was highest in week 1 p.p. (4.09%) and decreased to 3.03% in week 4 p.p.. Protein content decreased significantly in restricted cows from initially 3.37% to a mean value of 3.19% in period 2. In week 1 of realimentation, restricted cows had a lower milk protein percentage (3.33 vs. 3.39%; $P < 0.05$), but recovered completely thereafter.

Body weight and body condition parameters
BW decreased after parturition from 668 kg (week 1 p.p.) to 647 kg (week 4 p.p.). In period 2, feed-restricted cows showed a lower BW than control animals (627 vs. 655 kg; $P < 0.05$). During the realimentation period, restricted cows gained BW and were equal to control cows from week 2 onwards. BCS declined from 3.29 (week 1 p.p.) to 2.99 (week 8 p.p.). In period 2, feed-restricted cows showed a lower BCS than control animals (2.79 vs. 3.02; $P < 0.05$). During the realimentation period, BCS increased for restricted cows to the level of control cows. Backfat thickness and the muscle diameter of the longissimus dorsi muscle decreased after parturition from 4.6 and 45.5 mm (week 1 p.p.) to 2.7 and 38.1 mm (week 8 p.p.). In period 2, feed-restricted cows showed a lower backfat thickness and a lower muscle diameter than control animals (1.8 vs. 2.6 mm; 37.3 vs. 40.0 mm, respectively; $P < 0.05$). During the realimentation period, only muscle diameter fully recovered in restricted cows. Backfat thickness increased during period 3, but did not reach the level of control cows.

Plasma metabolites
Plasma glucose concentration had a nadir in week 2 p.p. (3.30 mmol/L) and increased to 4.13 mmol/L in week 12 p.p.. For restricted cows, glucose concentration was lower (3.85 vs. 4.06 mmol/L; $P < 0.05$) in period 2 and reached the level of control cows again in week 4 of period 3. NEFA concentration was highest in period 1 in week 2 p.p. (0.90 ± 0.06 mmol/L) and decreased to 0.13 mmol/L in week 12 p.p.. Restricted cows had higher values of NEFA in period 2 (0.23 mmol/L) than control cows (0.14 mmol/L; $P < 0.05$). In period 3, there were no more detectable differences for NEFA concentration between the groups. Plasma BHBA increased from 0.70 mmol/L (week 1 p.p.) to a maximum in week 3 p.p. (0.98 mmol/L).

Thereafter values declined to 0.50 mmol/L from week 7-12 p.p.. In period 2, BHBA was slightly higher for restricted cows (0.62 vs. 0.52 mmol/L) and decreased in period 3 to the levels of control animals.

Endocrine parameters in plasma and hepatic gene expression

In period 1, plasma GH concentration was highest in week 1 p.p. (7.2 µg/L), whereas leptin, IGF-I and RQUICKI were lowest in week 1 and 2 p.p. (3.4 ng/mL, 65.6 ng/mL and 0.46, respectively). Plasma concentration of insulin showed a nadir in week 1 p.p. (3.3 µU/mL) and increased thereafter up to 7.1 µU/mL in week 12 p.p.. The concentration of T_3 and T_4 increased from 0.82 nmol/L and 41.7 nmol/L in week 1 p.p. up to 1.29 nmol/L and 64.6 nmol/L, respectively, in week 12 p.p.. During period 2, plasma GH was higher on average (6.0 vs. 5.0 µg/L), leptin (3.8 vs. 4.4 ng/mL) and IGF-I (99.0 vs. 120.8 ng/mL) were significantly lower in restricted compared to control cows ($P < 0.05$). RQUICKI was lower for restricted cows during period 2 compared to control cows (0.56 vs. 0.62; $P < 0.05$). Endocrine factors did not differ between the groups in the realimentation period. Feed-restriction and the subsequent realimentation period did not affect the concentration of insulin, T_3 and T_4.

Three days after parturition, hepatic mRNA abundance of GH receptor 1A (GHR 1A), IGF-I, IGF-I receptor (IGF-IR) and IGF binding protein-3 (IGFBP-3) were decreased, whereas mRNA of IGFBP-1 and -2 and insulin receptor (INSR) were up-regulated as compared to week 3 ante partum. At the end of the 3-week feed-restriction mRNA abundance of IGF-I, IGFBP-1, -2, -3 and INSR was increased compared to the control group ($P < 0.05$).

Milk fatty acid composition

During the NEB in early lactation, milk FA profile changed markedly up to week 12 p.p. and remained unchanged thereafter. Fatty acids up to C16 increased along with saturated fatty acids from week 1 p.p. up to week 12 p.p., whereas monounsaturated fatty acids, predominantly the proportion of C18:1,9c released from adipocytes decreased as NEB became less. During the deliberately induced NEB by feed-restriction milk FA profile showed a same directed pattern as during the NEB in early lactation, although changes were less intense for most fatty acids. The proportions of milk fatty acids changed rapidly within one week after initiation of feed-restriction and tended to adjust to the initial composition despite maintenance of a high NEB. C18:1,9c was increased significantly during the induced NEB indicating mobilization of a considerable amount of adipose tissue. Besides C18:1,9c as a single FA, changes in the summarized fatty acids (saturated, monounsaturated, de novo synthesized and preformed fatty acids) reflect energy status in dairy cows and indicate a NEB in terms of a constant feeding regimen.

The extent of changes in the studied parameters was smaller during the deliberately induced NEB compared to the NEB in early lactation, even though the induced NEB by feed-restriction was greater. The different adaptive reactions of dairy cows to an energy deficiency at two stages in lactation indicate the different levels of metabolic priority during the course of lactation.

Zusammenfassung

Homöorhese und Homöostase sind für Milchkühe unerlässlich bei der Anpassung an veränderte physiologische Gegebenheiten und Umweltbedingungen. Eine negative Energiebilanz (NEB) tritt gewöhnlich nach der Abkalbung bei Milchkühen auf, kann jedoch auch zu einem späteren Laktationszeitpunkt bei unzureichender Versorgung auftreten. Kühe müssen sich an eine NEB anpassen, um die Laktation und ihre Lebensfunktionen aufrecht zu erhalten. Ziel der vorliegenden Arbeit war es, die Anpassung von Leistungsparametern, des Stoffwechsels und des endokrinen Systems an eine laktationsbedingte und nutritiv ausgelöste negative Energiebilanz in Milchkühen zu untersuchen.

Fünfzig mehrkalbige Kühe der Rasse Holstein (3,2 ± 1,4 Laktationen) wurden in drei Abschnitten untersucht (Abschnitt 1 = Woche 3 ante partum bis einschließlich Woche 12 post partum; Abschnitt 2 = dreiwöchige Fütterungsrestriktion ab 98 ± 7 Laktationstagen mit einer Restriktions- und einer Kontrollgruppe zu je 25 Kühen; Abschnitt 3 = unmittelbar folgende achtwöchige Realimentationsphase der restriktiv gefütterten Gruppe). Während des gesamten Untersuchungszeitraums erhielten alle Kühe eine teilaufgewertete Mischration (PMR; basierend auf Mais- und Grassilage, Heu und Kraftfutter) mit Ausnahme der restriktiv gefütterten Kühe in Abschnitt 2 zur freien Aufnahme. In Abschnitt 2 wurde die NEB durch individuelle Begrenzung der Futtermenge und Energiedichte in der Ration ausgelöst. Bei einer Milchleistung über 21 kg/d wurde individuell zusätzliches Kraftfutter verabreicht, außer während der Restriktionsphase, in der die Menge auf 0,4 kg/d festgelegt wurde. Die Futteraufnahme und Milchleistung wurden täglich erfasst, die Lebendmasse wöchentlich. Blutproben wurden einmal pro Woche genommen, Milchproben zweimal wöchentlich. Die Entnahme von Leberbioptaten erfolgte in den Wochen 3 a.p., Woche 1 und 4 p.p. (Abschnitt 1) sowie in Woche 0 und 3 von Abschnitt 2. Aus der täglichen Futteraufnahme, dem Erhaltungsbedarf und der Milchmenge wurde die Energiebilanz für jedes Tier berechnet.

Futteraufnahme, Energiebilanz, Milchleistung und Milchinhaltsstoffe

Die Futteraufnahme stieg von 14,9 ± 0,2 kg/d (Woche 1 p.p.) auf über 22 kg/d in den Wochen 7 bis 12 von Abschnitt 1. Die NEB war mit -46,1 MJ NEL/d in Woche 1 p.p. am höchsten und deckte den Energiebedarf der Kühe nur zu 70%. Während Abschnitt 2 hatten die restriktiv gefütterten Kühe eine mittlere Futteraufnahme von 10,3 kg/d und deckten ihren Energiebedarf zu 51%, wohingegen die Kontrollkühe eine Futteraufnahme von 21,1 kg/d und eine Energiebilanz von 104% aufwiesen. In Woche 1 der Realimentation (Abschnitt 3) hatten die Kontrollkühe noch eine höhere Futteraufnahme als die restriktiven Kühe (20,4 vs. 18,7 kg/d; $P < 0,05$). Die Energiebilanz der restriktiv gefütterten Kühe wurde in Woche 2 von Abschnitt 3 positiv und erreichte bis zum Versuchsende 109% des berechneten Bedarfs (Kontrollkühe 108%). Die Milchleistung setzte in Woche 1 p.p. mit 27,5 ± 0,7 kg/d ein, erreichte in der sechsten Laktationswoche ein Maximum (39,5 ± 0,8 kg/d) und fiel auf 32,8 ± 0,8 kg/d in Woche 12 p.p.. Während Abschnitt 2 hatten die restriktiv gefütterten Kühe trotz der hohen nutritiv induzierten NEB nur eine geringfügig niedrigere Milchleistung (27,4 kg/d) im Vergleich zu den Kontrollkühen (30,5 kg/d; $P < 0,05$). Die Milchleistung der restriktiv gefütterten Kühe stieg in der ersten Woche von Abschnitt 3 und unterschied sich nicht vom Niveau der Kontrollkühe. Der Milchfettgehalt war in der ersten Laktationswoche am höchsten (5,48%) und fiel bis auf 4,00% in der siebten Woche p.p.. Innerhalb der ersten Woche von Abschnitt 2 stieg der Milchfettgehalt von 4,30 auf 4,63% ($P < 0,10$). Im restlichen Abschnitt 2 und in Abschnitt 3 waren keine Unterschiede zwischen den Gruppen festzustellen. Der Milcheiweißgehalt war in der ersten Woche p.p. am höchsten (4,09%) und fiel auf 3,03% in Woche 4 p.p.. Der Eiweißgehalt ging bei den restriktiv gefütterten Kühen von anfänglich 3,37% auf durchschnittlich 3,19% in Abschnitt 2 zurück. In der ersten Realimentationswoche zeigten die restriktiven Kühe einen geringeren Milcheiweißgehalt (3,33 vs. 3,39%; $P < 0,05$), der sich anschließend vollständig erholte.

Lebendmasse und Körperkonditionsparameter

Die Lebendmasse fiel nach der Abkalbung von 668 kg (Woche 1 p.p.) auf 647 kg in der vierten Laktationswoche. In Abschnitt 2 zeigten die restriktiv gefütterten Kühe eine geringere Lebendmasse als die Kontrollkühe (627 vs. 655 kg; $P < 0,05$). Während der Realimentation stieg die Lebendmasse der restriktiven Kühe und war mit den Kontrollkühen ab Woche 2 gleich auf. Der BCS nahm von 3,29 (Woche 1 p.p.) auf 2,99 (Woche 8 p.p.) ab. In Abschnitt 2 hatten die restriktiv gefütterten Kühe einen niedrigeren BCS als die Kontrolltiere (2,79 vs. 3,02; $P < 0,05$). Während der Realimentationsphase stieg der BCS der restriktiven Kühe wieder auf das Niveau der Kontrollkühe. Die Rückenfettdicke und der Rückenmuskeldurchmesser nahmen nach der Abkalbung von 4,6 und 45,5 mm in Woche 1 p.p. auf 2,7 bzw. 38,1 mm in Woche 8 p.p. ab. In Abschnitt 2 wiesen die restriktiven Kühe eine geringere Rückenfettdicke und einen geringeren Rückenmuskeldurchmesser im Vergleich zu den Kontrolltieren auf (1,8 vs. 2,6 mm bzw. 37,3 vs. 40,0 mm; $P < 0,05$). Während der Realimentationsperiode erholte sich nur der Muskeldurchmesser vollständig. Die Rückenfettdicke stieg in Abschnitt 3, erreichte jedoch nicht das Niveau der Kontrollkühe.

Stoffwechselparameter im Plasma

Die Plasma-Glukosekonzentration zeigte in der zweiten Laktationswoche einen Tiefpunkt (3,30 mmol/L) und stieg auf 4,13 mmol/L in der zwölften Laktationswoche. Bei den restriktiv gefütterten Kühen war die Glukosekonzentration in Abschnitt 2 niedriger (3,85 vs. 4,06 mmol/L; $P < 0,05$) und erreichte das Niveau der Kontrollkühe wieder in der vierten Realimentationswoche. Die Konzentration an freien Fettsäuren war in der zweiten Laktationswoche am höchsten (0,90 ± 0,06 mmol/L) und fiel auf 0,13 mmol/L in der Woche 12 p.p.. Die restriktiv gefütterten Kühe hatten in Abschnitt 2 höhere NEFA Werte (0,23 mmol/L) als die Kontrollkühe (0,14 mmol/L; $P < 0,05$). In Abschnitt 3 waren keine Unterschiede in der NEFA-Konzentration zwischen den Gruppen festzustellen. Die Plasmakonzentration von BHBA stieg von 0,70mmol/L in Woche 1 p.p. auf ein Maximum von 0,98 mmol/L in der dritten Laktationswoche. Die Werte für BHBA fielen im Anschluss auf 0,50 mmol/L in den Wochen 7 bis 12 p.p.. In Abschnitt 2 war die BHBA-Konzentration für die restriktiven Kühe etwas höher (0,62 vs. 0,52 mmol/L) und fiel in Abschnitt 3 auf das Niveau der Kontrolltiere.

Endokrine Faktoren im Plasma und Genexpressionen in der Leber

In Abschnitt 1 war die Plasmakonzentration von Wachstumshormon (GH) in der ersten Laktationswoche am höchsten (7,2 µg/L), während die Konzentrationen von Leptin, des insulinähnlichen Wachstumsfaktors-I (IGF-I) und des revised quantitative insulin sensitivity check index (RQUICKI) in der ersten und zweiten Woche p.p. am niedrigsten waren (3,4 ng/mL, 65,6 ng/mL bzw. 0,46). Die Insulinkonzentration im Plasma zeigte einen Tiefpunkt in Woche 1 p.p. (3,3 µU/mL) und stieg anschließend auf 7,1 µU/mL in Woche 12 p.p.. Die Konzentration von T_3 und T_4 stieg von 0,82 nmol/L bzw. 41,7 nmol/L in Woche 1 p.p. auf 1,29 bzw. 64,6 nmol/L in der zwölften Laktationswoche. Während Abschnitt 2 war die GH-Konzentration im Mittel höher (6,0 vs. 5,0 µg/L), von Leptin (3,8 vs. 4,4 ng/mL) und IGF-I (99,0 vs. 120,8 ng/mL) dagegen bei den restriktiven Kühen signifikant niedriger im Vergleich zu den Kontrollkühen ($P < 0,05$). RQUICKI war für die restriktive Gruppe im Vergleich zur Kontrolle während Abschnitt 2 niedriger (0,56 vs. 0,62; $P < 0,05$). In der Realimentation waren keine Unterschiede in den endokrinen Faktoren zwischen den Gruppen festzustellen. Die Fütterungsrestriktion und die folgende Realimentierung hatten keinen Einfluss auf die Konzentration von Insulin, T_3 und T_4.

Am Tag 3 p.p. war die mRNA Menge von GH Rezeptor 1A (GHR 1A), IGF-I, IGF-I Rezeptor (IGF-IR) und IGF-Bindungsprotein-3 (IGFBP-3) reduziert, wohingegen die

Expressionen von IGFBP-1, -2 sowie des Insulinrezeptors (INSR) im Vergleich zur Woche 3 ante partum hochreguliert waren. Am Ende der dreiwöchigen Restriktionsphase waren die Genexpressionen von IGF-I, IGFBP-1, -2, -3 und INSR gegenüber der Kontrollgruppe erhöht ($P < 0,05$).

Milchfettsäuremuster

Während der NEB in der Frühlaktation zeigte das Milchfettsäuremuster bis zu 12. Laktationswoche deutliche Veränderungen und blieb anschließend unverändert. Die Fettsäuren (FS) bis C16 stiegen zusammen mit den gesättigten FS von der ersten bis zur zwölften Laktationswoche, während der Anteil der einfach ungesättigten FS, insbesondere C18:1,9c aus den Adipozyten, mit abnehmender NEB zurückging. Während der durch Fütterungsrestriktion induzierten NEB zeigte das Milchfettsäuremuster gleichgerichtete Änderungen wie während der NEB in der Frühlaktation, obwohl das Ausmaß der Veränderungen für die meisten FS weniger groß war. Die Anteile der FS änderten sich rasch innerhalb der ersten Restriktionswoche und tendierten zur Angleichung an die ursprüngliche Zusammensetzung trotz Aufrechterhaltung einer hohen NEB. Der Anteil von C18:1,9c stieg deutlich während der Restriktionsphase an, was auf die Mobilisierung von Fettgewebe hinweist. Neben C18:1,9c als Einzelfettsäure spiegelten die Veränderungen in der Summe der gesättigten FS, der einfach ungesättigten FS, der neusynthetisierten und vorgeformten FS den Energiestatus von Milchkühen wider und deuteten bei gleichbleibendem Fütterungsregime auf eine NEB hin.

Das Ausmaß der Auswirkungen in den untersuchten Parametern war während der induzierten NEB geringer im Vergleich zur NEB in der Frühlaktation, obgleich die durch Fütterungsrestriktion induzierte NEB größer war. Die unterschiedlichen Anpassungsreaktionen von Milchkühen an ein Energiedefizit zu zwei Laktationszeitpunkten zeigen die verschiedenen Stufen der Stoffwechselpriorität während des Laktationsverlaufs.

1. Introduction

World's total milk production of round 697 million tons in 2009 was covered to 83% by cow's milk (FAO, 2011). Compared to 1979, the world wide milk production of dairy cows was increased by 39% in 2009, whereas livestock of dairy cows increased only by 19% in the same period (FAO, 2011). These remarkable increases in milk yield during the past decades can be attributed to the intense genetic selection in high-yielding breeds such as Holstein-Friesians.

At the onset of lactation, nutritional and energetic requirements can increase 4-fold in high-yielding dairy cows within one day relative to late pregnancy (Carriquiry et al., 2009). Veerkamp et al. (2000) indicated that the increase in genetic merit for feed intake did not parallel that for milk yield in dairy cows compared to suckling cows. The lag in feed intake behind the faster increasing energy output by milk production affects energy status markedly leading to a negative energy balance (NEB) that can last up to week 14 of lactation (Ingvartsen and Andersen, 2000; NRC, 2001). Energy balance (EB) is defined as the difference between the energy uptake by feed and the energy output required for maintenance, growth, pregnancy and lactation (Grummer, 2007). A more adequate term that Butler et al. (2003) proposed might be 'lactational' or 'lactation-induced NEB', as this situation occurs naturally after calving and depends on the amount of milk yield and simultaneous dry matter intake (DMI) in dairy cows. The energy and nutrient shortfall in early lactation is met by mobilization of body reserves, predominantly localized in adipose and muscle tissue, and by shifting the pattern of nutrients used by non-mammary tissues (Bauman and Currie, 1980). The priority of milk production and nutrient partitioning towards the mammary gland after parturition is expressed by increased milk yield despite the lactational NEB.

The mobilization of endogenous reserves accreted during the preceding late lactation and pregnancy can be excessive and may result in health disorders (Bertoni et al., 2009) expressed in an increase in incidence and severity of metabolic disorders. Energy status has been indicated as an important factor involved. Epidemiological studies found a NEB directly or indirectly via milk yield related to fatty liver, ketosis (Grummer, 1993), infectious diseases (Collard et al., 2000) and reduced reproductive performance (Lopez et al., 2004).

A NEB may occur later in lactation during insufficient supply and quality of feed. Due to the seasonal nature of pasture growth, it is almost inevitable that dairy cows are subjected to periods of undernutrition when they are completely dependent on grassland for energy and nutrient supply (Trigg et al., 1979). Furthermore, a NEB may be existing during advanced lactation when feeding a TMR without taking into account the different performance levels and individual requirements of the cow. In this respect, energy density of the diet can be a limiting factor affecting performance. In these situations, dairy cows need to adapt to maintain homeostasis, which is defined as the property that regulates the endogenous environment and tends to maintain a stable physiological condition (Cannon, 1929; Bauman and Currie, 1980). The established lactation after the NEB in early lactation, i.e., in mid-lactation or in the so-called production phase of lactation, represents such a stable physiological equilibrium during which the metabolic priority of the mammary gland no longer exists. An induced NEB at this stage of lactation resulted in a reduced milk yield with elevated plasma NEFA concentration (Carlson et al., 2006).

Mechanisms coordinating adaptations to the lactation-induced NEB have been the subject of numerous investigations over the last three decades (Bauman and Currie, 1980; Bell and Bauman, 1997; Vernon and Pond, 1997). Boisclair et al. (2006) suppose motivation in research two major considerations for these efforts. First, dairy cows offer a unique model to study metabolic changes during the transition from an energy-sufficient to an energy-insufficient state (late pregnancy vs. early lactation). Second, failure in one or more metabolic adaptations is thought to underlie a major portion of the increased susceptibility of early lactating dairy cows to metabolic diseases and associated disorders (Goff and Horst, 1997; Ingvartsen et al., 2003).

Performance and physiological reactions in dairy cows are influenced by homeorhetic and homeostatic control. Studies of homeorhetic and homeostatic control in early and mid-lactation are scarce. Therefore, the differential adaptation of performance, metabolism and endocrine systems to the lactational and a nutrition induced negative energy balance at around 100 days in milk (DIM) in dairy cows is subject of this study.

Results out of the present study are thought to improve basic knowledge of physiology of high-yielding dairy cows during energy deficient situations and to be integrated as a part of the basis for decision in the ongoing genetic selection process.

2. Material and Methods

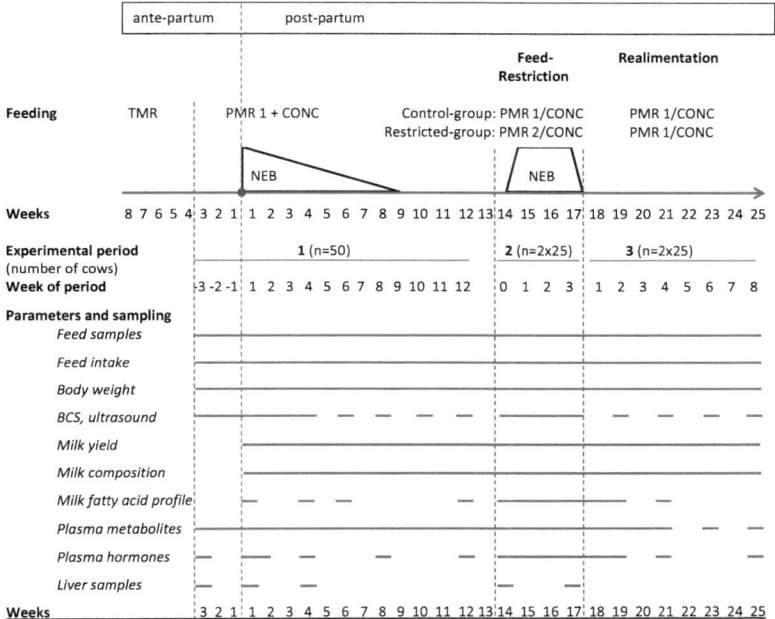

Figure 1. Experimental design and sampling schedule.

2.1 Experimental design, animals and housing

The animal trial was conducted at the Agricultural Experimental Unit Hirschau of the Technische Universität München under supervision of the responsible state department for animal welfare affairs. Fifty multiparous Holstein dairy cows (3.2 ± 1.4 parities, mean ± SD) out of a herd of 100 were studied from week 3 ante partum (a.p.) to about week 25 post partum (p.p.) in three experimental periods (Figure 1). Cows were dried off 8 weeks before expected calving and kept separately until week 4 a.p.. From week 3 a.p. onwards, dry cows were integrated into the lactating herd that was housed in a free stall barn. From 10 days before the expected calving until day 5 p.p. (end of the colostral period), animals were fed individually in calving pens with straw bedding. Thereafter, cows joined the lactating herd in the free stall barn with lying cubicles until the end of the study.

Experimental **period 1** reached from week 3 a.p. up to week 12 p.p., where all cows were treated as one group (see Figure 1). In **period 2** at around 100 DIM (week 14 p.p.), cows were divided equally to either a control (C; n=25) or a restriction group (R; n=25) according to the extent of NEB the cows experienced in period 1 with feed-restriction for 3 weeks (weeks 15 to 17 p.p., Figure 1). The week before feed-restriction was classified as week 0, where all cows were treated as one group. After 3 weeks of the deliberately induced NEB, **period 3** (weeks 18 to 25 p.p., Figure 1) started, where R-cows were (re)fed similarly as C-cows.

2.2 Feeding regimen

During the dry period from week 8 a.p. to 4 a.p., cows received a low energy, straw rich total mixed ration (TMR) for ad libitum intake. Dietary composition and the nutrient value of the TMR are given in Tables 1 and 2. Animals in period 1 (beginning in week 3 a.p. onwards) received a partial mixed ration 1 (PMR 1; Tables 1, 2) for ad libitum intake with separate and limited intake of concentrate. The PMR 1 was calculated to meet the demands for energy and protein of a cow (650 kg BW) producing 21 kg milk/d with an assumed DMI of 16 kg DM/d.

Table 1. Composition of the experimental diets and the concentrate.

	TMR	PMR 1	PMR 2	CONC
Components (% in DM)				
Grass silage		33.7	21.8	
Corn silage	38.6	44.9	29.1	
Hay		6.5	39.4	
Straw	44.6			
Barley				14.9
Corn kernels				24.8
Wheat				21.8
Soybean meal				20.1
Rapeseed meal	15.5			
Dried sugar beet pulp with molasses				15.2
Vitamin-mineral-premix	1.3^1			2.1^2
Limestone				1.1
Concentrate^3		14.9	9.7	
Total (%)	**100.0**	**100.0**	**100.0**	**100.0**

[1] Vitamin-mineral-premix for dry cows
[2] Vitamin-mineral-premix for lactating dairy cows
[3] Concentrate applied to PMR 1 and PMR 2 consisting of 7.9% barley, 24.7% wheat, 60.0% soybean meal 4.1% vitamin-mineral-premix for lactating cows, 2.3% limestone and 1.0% salt.

The PMR 1 was given once daily at 0930 h. Feeding troughs for recording individual PMR intake were connected to electronic balances. In addition to PMR 1, concentrate (CONC; Tables 1, 2) was fed at 0.7 kg DM/d until parturition and at 1.3 kg DM/d for the first 5 days of lactation. Up to day 42 p.p., CONC was increased from 1.8 kg DM/d up to 8.9 kg DM/d. Thereafter, CONC was fed according to individual extra requirements for milk production when daily milk yield was above 21 kg. The CONC was offered in transponder access feeding stations by an automatic feeding program (DeLaval Alpro, Glinde, Germany).

At the start of period 2, R-cows received PMR 1 with additional hay to reduce the energy content (PMR 2; Tables 1, 2). Furthermore, CONC was limited to 0.4 kg DM/d for all R-cows during period 2. The amount of PMR 2 was limited in each week of period 2 to maintain an energy deficiency of a least 30% of the calculated requirements. As a consequence of feed restriction, the protein supply was reduced correspondingly. The C-cows were maintained on PMR 1 ad libitum as in period 1.

Table 2. Nutrient values of experimental diets and concentrate.

	TMR	PMR 1	PMR 2	CONC
Nutrient values				
MJ NE_L/kg DM[1]	5.32 ± 0.08	6.53 ± 0.08	6.24 ± 0.05	7.96 ± 0.04
Crude fiber (g/kg DM)	296 ± 24	214 ± 23	251 ± 27	62 ± 5
Crude ash (g/kg DM)	66 ± 10	76 ± 9	75 ± 18	76 ± 13
Crude fat (g/kg DM)	22 ± 6	32 ± 6	28 ± 6	24 ± 6
CP (g/kg DM)	104 ± 16	146 ± 8	138 ± 38	216 ± 38
NDF (g/kg DM)	538	431	529	184
ADF (g/kg DM)	377	254	313	84.1
ADL (g/kg DM)	40.2	23.6	32.4	3.9
NFC (g/kg DM)[1,2]	270	316	230	500
Available CP (g/kg DM)[1]	118 ± 7	143 ± 20	137 ± 29	172 ± 12
RNB (g/kg DM)[4]	-1.5 ± 0.6	0.9 ± 1.0	0.2 ± 1.9	2.4 ± 0.4

[1] Calculated values.
[2] Nonfiber carbohydrates calculated by difference: 100 − (% CP + % NDF + % crude fat + % crude ash).

In period 3, R-cows had free access to PMR 1 until the end of the study. The CONC was set from 0.4 to 4.5 kg DM/d (= mean value of C-group) in week 1 of realimentation. During the rest of period 3, CONC was adapted weekly for all animals as described above. For each cow daily DMI (PMR and CONC) was recorded continuously. Changes of the diets were carried out all at once within a day. All animals had free access to fresh water.

2.3 Analysis of feed samples and determination of energy and protein balance

Samples of forages (grass silage, corn silage) provided with TMR, PMR 1, PMR 2 and the CONC were collected weekly. Samples of TMR, PMR 1 and 2 were obtained twice per week. For analysis of DM, fresh feeds were weighed, dried for 24 h at 60 °C and reweighed. Samples were milled (Brabender, Duisburg, Germany; filter width 1.1 mm) and mixed together into 2-week sample pools (except CONC 4-week sample pooled) for further analyses. Feed samples were analyzed for crude ash, crude fiber and crude fat according to Weende analysis (Naumann et al., 2000). Crude protein (CP; N x 6.25) content was determined by the Dumas method. The nutrient values of the forages used in the experimental diets and the concentrate are shown in Table 3.

Table 3. Nutrient value of forages used in the experimental diets and the concentrate.

Components	MJ NE_L/kg DM	Crude fiber	Crude ash	Crude fat	Crude protein	ACP	RNB
				g/kg DM			
Grass silage	5.82 ± 0.23	250 ± 24	114 ± 27	40 ± 6	170 ± 18	133 ± 6	5.9 ± 2.3
Corn silage	6.77 ± 0.05	177 ± 12	32 ± 5	35 ± 4	78 ± 7	134 ± 2	-9.0 ± 0.8
Hay	5.73 ± 0.05	333 ± 34	66 ± 14	14 ± 4	93 ± 35	122 ± 8	-4.6 ± 4.4
Straw	3.59 ± 0.12	439 ± 28	63 ± 9	12 ± 3	49 ± 9	79 ± 3	-5.4 ± 1.0
Barley	7.94 ± 0.04	78 ± 18	29 ± 4	20 ± 5	119 ± 9	158 ± 2	-6.2 ± 1.1
Corn kernels	8.41 ± 0.14	46 ± 2	24 ± 11	58 ± 17	99 ± 6	161 ± 3	-10.1 ± 0.7
Wheat	8.46 ± 0.02	34 ± 5	19 ± 1	11 ± 1	140 ± 7	169 ± 2	-4.8 ± 0.9
Soybean meal	8.57 ± 0.09	88 ± 13	75 ± 7	18 ± 8	493 ± 14	246 ± 4	39.7 ± 1.7
Rapeseed meal	7.12 ± 0.26	147 ± 7	119 ± 29	24 ± 7	367 ± 7	200 ± 6	27.7 ± 0.5
Dried sugar beet pulp with molasses	7.43 ± 0.03	158 ± 6	69 ± 3	5 ± 4	98 ± 5	146 ± 1	-7.6 ± 0.6

NDF, ADF and lignin (ADL) were analyzed for TMR, PMR 1, PMR 2 and CONC according to Naumann et al. (2000) (Table 2). The FA composition of PMR 1, PMR 2 and CONC was determined using FA methyl esters (FAME) prepared by transesterification with trimethylsulfonium hydroxide (TMSH). FAMEs were analyzed using gas chromatography (GC 6890, Agilent Technologies, Waldbronn, Germany) to determine isomer distribution patterns. Quantification of FA was performed with the chromatography software Chromeleon 6.8 (Dionex, Sunnyvale, California, USA). Table 4 shows the FA composition of PMR 1, PMR 2 and CONC.

Table 4. Fatty acid composition of the experimental diets and the concentrate.

	PMR 1	PMR 2	CONC
FA (g/100g FAME)			
12:0	0.10	0.14	< 0.05
14:0	0.50	0.65	0.19
15:0	0.10	0.20	0.14
16:0	16.93	19.97	27.80
16:1,9c	0.28	0.39	0.16
17:0	0.18	0.25	0.20
17:1,10c	0.13	0.18	0.05
18:0	2.72	2.57	4.18
18:1,9t	0.10	0.12	0.08
18:1,9c	15.90	13.32	20.49
18:1,11c	1.02	0.92	1.47
18:2,9c,12c	37.57	33.36	38.70
18:3,9c,12c,15c	18.59	21.33	2.66
20:0	0.55	0.55	0.52
20:1,11c	0.21	0.16	0.34
22:0	0.66	0.75	0.56
23:0	0.16	0.28	0.22
24:0	0.78	0.87	0.73
SFA	22.68	26.23	34.55
MUFA	17.54	14.97	22.51
PUFA	56.16	54.69	41.36
trans FA	0.10	0.12	0.08
CLA	< 0.05	< 0.05	< 0.05
not identified peaks	3.52	4.00	1.50

Calculations for energy and protein supply followed the recommendations of the German Society of Nutrition Physiology (GfE, 2001). Net energy (NEL) and available CP at the duodenum (ACP), and the ruminal nitrogen balance (RNB) of the forages used were calculated out of the results from the Weende analysis according to the German Society of Nutrition Physiology (GfE, 2001) considering the digestibilities of the respective crude nutrients tabulated in DLG (1997). The energy content of TMR, PMR 1, PMR 2 and CONC was calculated by multiplying the energy density of the single components (Table 3) with their relative proportion in the diets (Table 1). The energy balance was calculated for each cow individually as the difference between energy intake through feed and energy requirements for maintenance, pregnancy and milk production. Energy intake was determined by multiplying average weekly DMI of PMR 1 and 2 and CONC with the corresponding energy content. Energy requirements for maintenance and pregnancy were quantified according to GfE (2001) by using the average weekly BW of the animal. Milk energy output resulted from milk yield, content of mean fat, protein and lactose of weekly pooled samples according to GfE (2001). Mobilization or deposition of body tissue, in cases of negative and positive energy balance, respectively, were not accounted for in the calculations.

The balance of ACP was calculated for each cow individually as the difference between ACP intake through feed and ACP requirement for maintenance, pregnancy and milk production according to GfE (2001).

2.4 Milk samples and analysis

Cows were milked twice daily in a 2 x 6 herringbone milking parlor (DeLaval) at 0500 and 1500 h. Daily milk yield was recorded electronically. During the colostrum period (day 1 to 5 p.p.) or treatments of mastitis, milk was separated and manually weighed. Milk samples (about 50 mL) were collected beginning at 3 d p.p. twice weekly on two consecutive milkings each (Monday p.m., Tuesday a.m., Thursday p.m., and Friday a.m.). Average fat, protein and lactose concentrations were determined by an infrared-spectrophotometer (MilcoScan-FT-6000, Foss Analytical A/S, Hillerød, Denmark) in the laboratory of the Milchprüfring Bayern e.V. (Wolnzach, Germany).

For determination of milk fatty acid (FA) composition, milk samples from two consecutive milkings (Monday p.m. and Tuesday a.m.) were stored at -20 °C until analysis. Milk FA composition was determined in samples of week 1, 4, 6 and 12 p.p. of period 1, weekly during period 2 and in week 1, 2 and 4 of period 3. Period 2 and 3 elongate the period p.p. over the weeks 1 to 12 (period 1) up to week 21 p.p. (Figure 1). Milk fat was extracted according to Bligh and Dyer (1959), modified by Hallermayer (1976). Analysis of FA composition in milk samples was determined as described for feed samples in chapter 2.3. Data of the FA composition in milk are given as weighted means of the separate milkings within the respective weeks.

2.5 Body weight and body condition parameters

The BW was recorded automatically on electronic scales mounted in the concentrate feeders. Body condition was scored according to Edmonson et al. (1989) on a scale between 1 and 5 (1 = thin, 5 = obese). Simultaneously, B-mode ultrasonographic measurements of the longissimus dorsi muscle diameter (MD) and backfat thickness (BFT) were performed with a 5 MHz (3.5-7.5 MHz) linear probe (Toshiba PLB 508M, Toshiba Medical Instruments, Tokyo, Japan) on the right side at the fifth loin vertebra. Positions were clipped and fluid paraffin oil was added to couple the ultrasound probe to the skin as described in Bruckmaier et al. (1998a). The MD and BFT were evaluated graphically according to Bruckmaier et al. (1998b) using Adobe Photoshop CS4 Extended (Adobe Systems Incorporated, San Jose, CA). The BCS and ultrasonic measurements were performed at the same time by the same person.

2.6 Animal health

Occurrence of diseases and health disorders were detected by daily animal inspections. In situations of clinical signs or veterinary treatments, cases were documented and assigned to one of the classes "mastitis and other udder related problems", "reproductive tract and related problems", "claw problems" or "milk fever".

2.7 Blood samples and analysis

Blood samples were collected once weekly beginning in week 3 a.p. (Figure 1). Sampling was performed after milking prior to feeding between 0730 and 0900 h. Blood was collected via jugular puncture in two K_3EDTA-coated (2 x 9 mL) evacuated tubes (Greiner, Frickenhausen, Germany). Samples were cooled on wet-ice, centrifuged at 2,000 x g for 15 min, and the plasma was aliquoted in 1.5 mL Eppendorf-tubes, and stored at -20 °C until analysis for metabolites and hormones.

The concentrations of plasma glucose were measured using a kit from bioMérieux (Genève, Switzerland; no. 61269). Concentrations of nonesterified FA (NEFA) were analyzed with kit no. FA 115, and of beta-hydroxybutyrate (BHBA) with kit no. RB 1007 from Randox Laboratories Ltd. (Schwyz, Switzerland).

Plasma GH, IGF-I, insulin, 3,5,3'-trijodthyronine (T_3) and thyroxine (T_4) were measured by radioimmunoassay as described by Vicari et al. (2008). Plasma leptin was measured by radioimmunoassay with an antibody against bovine leptin kindly provided by Prof. Helga Sauerwein, University of Bonn, Germany (Sauerwein et al., 2004).

As a measure of insulin sensitivity, the "revised quantitative insulin sensitivity check index" – RQUICKI – was calculated. The RQUICKI is based on the concentrations of plasma glucose, NEFA and insulin and may be an instrument to estimate insulin sensitivity in dairy cows (Holtenius and Holtenius, 2007). The RQUICKI is estimated according to the equation given by Perseghin et al. (2001, cited in: Holtenius and Holtenius, 2007):

$$RQUICKI = 1 / [\log (glucose) + \log (insulin) + \log (NEFA)].$$

2.8 Liver samples and analysis

Liver samples were obtained by blind percutaneous needle biopsy (14 G x 152 mm, Dispomed Witt oHG, Gelnhausen, Germany) under local anesthesia after blood sampling as described by van Dorland et al. (2009) in week 3 a.p., week 1 p.p. (on day 3 p.p.), week 4 p.p. (period 1), before feed-restriction in week 0 and week 3 of period 2 (Figure 1). Liver tissue (40 to 60 mg) was directly put into a RNA stabilization reagent (RNAlater, Ambion, Applied Biosystems Business, Austin, TX, USA), and kept at +4 °C for 24 h, and thereafter stored at -20 °C until analyzed. Total RNA was isolated from liver tissue using peqGOLD TriFast (PEQLAB Biotechnologie GmbH, Erlangen, Germany) according to the manufacturer`s instructions. The yield and purity of total RNA were detected by spectrophotometer with a BioPhotometer (Vaudaux-Eppendorf, Basel, Switzerland). RNA integrity was verified by the OD260/OD280 absorption ratio, which was between 1.7 and 2.1 for all samples.

For reverse transcription, 1 µg of extracted total RNA was reverse transcribed with 200 U Moleney Murine Leukemia Virus Reverse Transcriptase RNAase H Minus, Point Mutant (Promega Corporation, Madison, WI, USA) using 100 pmol random hexamer primers (Invitrogen, Leek, the Netherlands). The obtained cDNA was diluted to a final concentration of 25 ng/µL. The genes selected to measure the expression from the somatotropic axis are described in Table 5. The PCR quantification was performed with the Rotor-Gene 6000 (Corbett Research, Sydney, Australia), using the software version 1.7.40. Fluorescence take off was calculated with the "second derivative maximum" program option. A master-mix of the following reaction components was prepared: 1.8 µL DEPC-water, 1.0 µL forward primer (5 pmol), 1.0 µL reverse primer (5 pmol), 0.2 µL 50x SYBR-Green (20 pmol) and 5.0 µL 2x SensiMix (1 mM MgCl2) (2x SensiMix NoRef DNA Kit). In total, 9 µL of master-mix and 1 µL of sample volume, containing 25 ng of cDNA, were used. The following three-step PCR-program was used: denaturation for 10 min at 95 °C, 40 cycles of amplification (each consisting of 15 s at 95 °C, the primer specific annealing temperature for 30 s (see Table 5), and extension at 72 °C for 20 s and quantification of fluorescence), and finally a melting curve program (60 to 95 °C). The mRNA abundance of target genes was calculated relative to the mean mRNA abundance of the reference genes GAPDH and UBQ. Detailed information of the primers used for GAPDH and UBQ in given in Table 5. The mRNA levels of the housekeeping genes were stable across the time points (17.7 ± 0.1, 17.6 ± 0.2, 17.4 ± 0.2, 17.0 ± 0.1 and 17.1 ± 0.3 on week 3 a.p., week 1 p.p., week 4 p.p. (period 1), week 0 and 3 of period 2, respectively).

Table 5. PCR primer information, annealing temperature, and the PCR product length for genes analyzed in liver samples.

Gene[1]		Sequence 5'-3'	GeneBank accession no.	Annealing temperature (°C)	Length
GAPDH	for	TACATGGTCTACATGTTCCAGTATG	NM 001034034	60	439 bp
	rev	CAGTCTTCTGGGTGGCAGTGATG			
GHR 1A	for	CCAGTTTCCATGGTTCTTAATTAT	NM_176608.1	60	138 bp
	rev	TTCCTTTAATCTTTGGAACTGG			
IGF-I	for	TCGCATCTCTTCTATCTGGCCCTGT	NM_001077828.1	60	240 bp
	rev	GCAGTACATCTCCAGCCTCCTCAGA			
IGF-IR	for	TTAAAATGGCCAGAACCTGAG	XM_002696504.1	60	314 bp
	rev	ATTATAACCAAGCCTCCCAC			
IGFBP-1	for	TCAAGAAGTGGAAGGAGCCCT	NM_174554.2	60	127 bp
	rev	AATCCATTCTTGTTGCAGTTT			
IGFBP-2	for	CACCGGCAGATGGGCAA	NM_174555	60	136 bp
	rev	GAAGGCGCATGGTGGTGGAGAT			
IGFBP-3	for	ACAGACACCCAGAACTTCTCCTC	NM_174556.1	60	194 bp
	rev	GCTTCCTGCCCTTGGA			
INSR	for	TCCTCAAGGAGCTGGAGGAGT	XM_002688832.1	62	163 bp
	rev	GCTGCTGTCACATTCCCCA			
UBQ	for	AGATCCAGGATAAGGAAGGCAT	Z18245	62	198 bp
	rev	GCTCCACTTCCAGGGTGAT			

[1] GHR 1A, growth hormone receptor 1A; IGF-I, insulin-like growth factor-I; IGF-IR, IGF-I receptor; IGFBP, IGF binding protein; INSR, insulin receptor; UBQ, ubiquitin

2.9 Statistical evaluation

All data presented are means ± SEM. Statistical analysis was performed by use of the statistical software SAS, version 9.2 (SAS Institute, Cary, North Carolina, USA). Group differences over time were detected by the Bonferroni t-test (Fleiss, 1986). P-values < 0.05 were considered to be significant.

2.9.1 Performance, metabolic and health status data

For evaluation of the effects of the deliberately induced NEB by feed-restriction at 100 DIM (period 2), performance and metabolic data from the C- and R-group in period 2 and 3 were compared using a MIXED model (Cnaan et al., 1997). The model included week, group, parity and the week by group interaction as fixed effects. The area under the curve (AUC) (Hanley and McNeil, 1982) of the respective measures from week 1 to 12 p.p. was included additionally as a co-variable. The repeated subject was the individual cow.

The reactions of cows to the NEB in period 1 were compared with the reactions in period 2. This comparison was performed on the basis of AUC differences/week (Δ AUC/week) calculated for each period from the cows experiencing a NEB (period 1, week 1 to 3 p.p.; period 2, R-cows) and during the time they did not (period 1, week 1 a.p.; period 2, C-cows). The calculated Δ AUC/week for the measured traits in period 1 and 2 were statistically compared by using the MIXED procedure with experimental period and parity as fixed effects, and the individual cow as repeated subject.

For the statistical analysis of occurrence of health disorders, a one sample binomial test was used to evaluate the differences between R- and C-group.

2.9.2 Hormones and gene expression data

Changes over time within the R- and C-group were evaluated using obtained data on mRNA abundance and endocrine parameters at the respective time-points of liver biopsies in period 1 (week 3 a.p., week 1 p.p. (= day 3 p.p.), week 4 p.p.) and period 2 (week 0 and week 3). In the MIXED model time-point and parity were fixed effects.

In order to evaluate the effect of feed-restriction (period 2) on gene expression in liver, mRNA abundance (delta CT, $\log_2$; Livak and Schmittgen, 2001) in week 3 of period 2 was evaluated in a MIXED model including group and parity. Furthermore, the mRNA abundance of week 0 of period 2 was used as a co-variable and individual cow as repeated subject. To evaluate effects of feed-restriction on endocrine parameters for periods 2 and 3 (week 1 to 4), the areas under the curve (AUC) of R- and C-group were compared using the MIXED procedure of SAS. The model included group and parity as fixed effects. The AUC from week 8 p.p. until the beginning of period 2 (week 0) was included additionally as a co-variable. The repeated subject was the individual cow.

2.9.3 Milk FA and their relation to energy status

Relations between energy status and FA were expressed by the Pearson correlation coefficient. Changes in energy balance, feed intake, milk yield, milk composition and milk FA profile over time during lactation and feed-restriction with subsequent realimentation were evaluated by a mixed model with group and week as fixed effect.

14 Material and Methods

3. Results and Discussion

3.1 Adaptation of performance parameters to a NEB

Feed intake, milk yield, energy and ACP balance

In mammalian species, pregnancy and milk secretion have developed a high priority of energy and nutrient delivery during evolution (Bruckmaier and van Dorland, 2010). Feed intake is the crucial factor determining energy and nutrient supply according to the current requirements. Figure 2 shows the DMI in dairy cows of the present study.

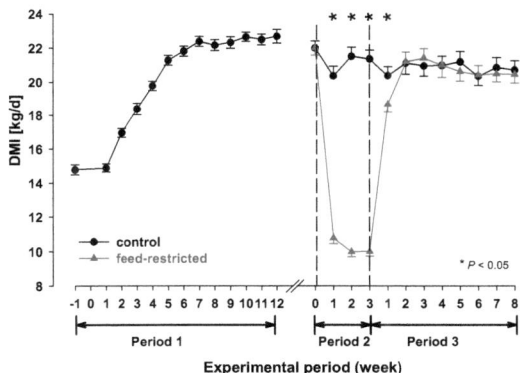

Figure 2. Dry matter intake (DMI; kg/d) in cows during the experimental periods. Differences between the groups in period 2 and 3 are indicated with * ($P < 0.05$).

In week 1 a.p., feed intake was 14.8 ± 0.3 kg/d and was not depressed during the periparturient period as reported by Grummer (1993). After parturition, the pattern of DMI followed previous findings (e.g., Ingvartsen and Andersen, 2000; Kessel et al., 2008). In week 1 p.p., total DMI started at 14.9 ± 0.6 kg/d, which was ~ 3 kg/d higher compared to the findings of Ingvartsen and Andersen (2000). Total DMI in the present study added up the ad libitum intake of the partial mixed ration (PMR) and the limited intake of concentrate. To avoid rumen acidosis, the amount of concentrate was increased slowly from 1.3 kg/d directly after parturition up to a maximum of 8.9 kg/d within 42 days. A plateau of DMI between 22 and 23 kg/d was reached from week 7 p.p. onwards (Figure 2).

When the intake of PMR and concentrate are multiplied with the respective energy density and content of ACP, total DMI mimics the energy and ACP intake of dairy cows. Figure 3 shows the energy intake of the cows during the study. In week 1 a.p., energy intake averaged

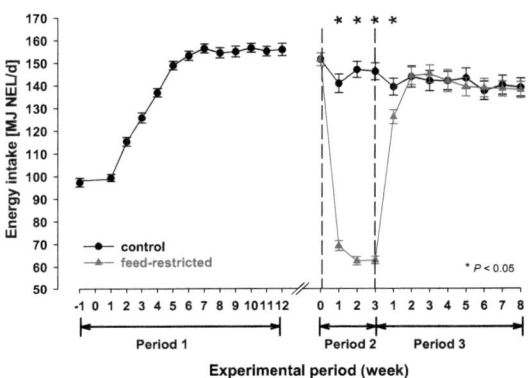

Figure 3. Energy intake (MJ NEL/d) in cows during the experimental periods. Differences between the groups in period 2 and 3 are indicated with * (P < 0.05).

97.4 ± 1.9 MJ NEL/d and increased along with DMI from 99.4 ± 1.5 MJ NEL/d in week 1 p.p. to a plateau of around 155 MJ NEL/d in week 7 onwards (Figure 3). In lactating dairy cows, energy output and ACP requirements are mainly determined by milk yield and milk solubles. In the present study, milk yield started with 27.5 ± 0.7 kg/d (mean milk yield of day 4 to 11 p.p.), reached a peak of 39.5 ± 0.8 kg/d in week 6 p.p., and declined to 33.7 ± 1.1 kg/d in week 12 p.p. (Figure 4). The time-point of peaking milk yield in week 6 p.p. complies with observations from the NRC (2001) and Piepenbrink et al. (2004), indicating milk production usually peaks between 4 and 8 weeks p.p. in dairy cows. The mammary gland has obviously the highest metabolic priority at the start of lactation. From an evolutionary point of view, it is reasonable that the priority of milk production for ruminants is highest after parturition during the colostral period and the following weeks when the offspring depends on milk as exclusive feed source (Morrill et al., 1981; Bruckmaier and van Dorland, 2010). Despite a negative energy balance in early lactation, the cow increases the daily milk yield at the risk of metabolic diseases up to the point during which the offspring gradually develops into a ruminant with the simultaneous decline in lactation curve.

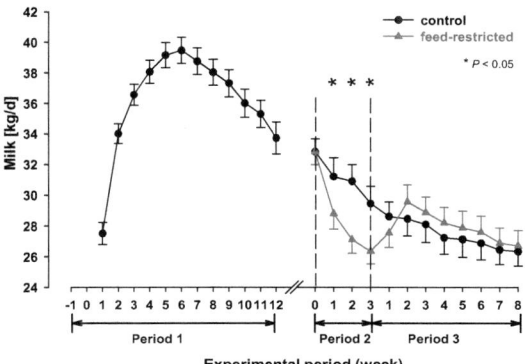

Figure 4. Milk yield (kg/d) in cows during the experimental periods. Differences between the groups in period 2 and 3 are indicated with * ($P < 0.05$).

Energy and ACP requirements were determined with equations including milk fat, protein and lactose content according to GfE (2001). Milk yield multiplied with the corresponding demands of energy and ACP per kg milk resulted in the total requirements of energy and ACP by lactation. The energy balance (Figure 5) and ACP balance (Figure 6) were calculated as the difference between intake via feed and requirements for maintenance, pregnancy and lactation. As milk production (Figure 4) rose faster after parturition than DMI (Figure 2), EB and the ACP balance were negative in early lactation.

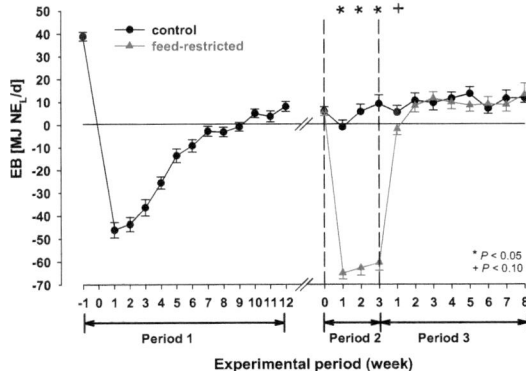

Figure 5. Energy balance (EB; MJ NEL/d) in cows during the experimental periods. Differences between the groups in period 2 and 3 are indicated with + ($P < 0.10$) and * ($P < 0.05$).

EB dropped from 38.9 ± 1.8 MJ NEL/d in week 1 a.p. within one week to a nadir of -46.1 ± 3.4 MJ NEL/d in week 1 p.p. (Figure 5) that covered energy demands by 70 ± 2%. With increasing energy intake in the following weeks, the NEB diminished and turned positive in week 9 p.p.. The occurrence of a NEB in early lactating cows was found in many studies, e.g., Ingvartsen and Andersen (2000), Jorritsma et al. (2003) and Kessel et al. (2008). Its duration may last up to 14 weeks p.p. (NRC, 2001). At the end of period 1 (week 12 p.p.), EB averaged 8.0 ± 2.2 MJ NEL/d that covered energy requirements by 106 ± 2% (Figure 5).

According to EB, the balance of ACP dropped as sudden after parturition from +895 g/d to a nadir of -1,002 g/d in week 1 p.p. (Figure 6). With increasing DMI, the negative ACP balance became less and turned positive on average in week 10 p.p. (28 ± 50 g/d; Figure 6).

The NEB starting around 100 DIM in period 2 was induced by feed-restriction. In order to achieve and to maintain a NEB of at least 30% of the calculated energy requirements for three weeks, the amount of PMR and concentrate was limited for restricted cows. Additionally, hay was mixed into the PMR to reduce its energy density whilst achieving a sufficient rumen filling. Due to the limited feed available for feed-restricted cows, their DMI dropped from 22.0 ± 0.4 kg/d before feed-restriction in week 0 within one week to 10.8 ± 0.3 kg/d and remained at this level during the three weeks of period 2 (Figure 2). For the control group, DMI was stable between 20 and 21 kg/d until the end of the study. In the realimentation period (period 3) following feed-restriction, restricted cows underwent the same feeding regimen as control cows. DMI increased to 18.7 ± 0.5 kg/d in week 1 of realimentation for restricted cows, which was ~ 1.5 kg/d lower compared to control cows (20.4 ± 0.5 kg/d, $P < 0.05$). From week 2 until the end of the study, no more differences in feed intake between the two groups were found (Figure 2). According to the DMI of restricted cows, energy intake averaged 65.0 ± 1.9 MJ NEL/d during period 2 and rapidly increased to the level of control cows of around 140 MJ NEL/d within two weeks of the following realimentation period (Figure 3).

According to the DMI and hereby energy intake, EB turned negative in feed-restricted cows within the first week of period 2 at a value of -65.0 ± 2.6 MJ NEL/d that covered only 51 ± 2% of their energy requirements. On average, the nutrition induced NEB remained at a level of -63 MJ NEL/d throughout the feed-restriction period (Figure 5). Thus, the extent of the NEB induced by feed-restriction in period 2 was greater compared to the lactation-induced NEB. In the first week of realimentation, EB in energy-restricted cows was still slightly negative (-1.7 ± 2.6 MJ NEL/d) and turned positive again in the following weeks of period 3

(Figure 5). As expected, EB in C-cows was positive throughout experimental periods 2 and 3 (Figure 5).

ACP balance dropped within one week from initially 99 ± 46 g/d to -1,247 ± 52 g/d in the first week of the feed-restriction period and stayed at the level of around -1,200 g/d during period 2 (Figure 6). In the subsequent realimentation (period 3), the balance of ACP turned immediately positive and rose up to +308 ± 107 g/d at the end of period 3 (Figure 6).

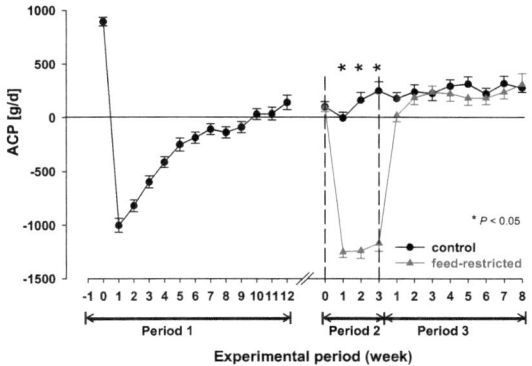

Figure 6. Available crude protein balance (ACP; g/d) in cows during the experimental periods. Differences between the groups in period 2 and 3 are indicated with * ($P < 0.05$).

During feed-restriction, milk yield decreased from 32.8 ± 0.8 kg/d (week 0 of period 2) to 28.8 ± 1.0 kg/d for restricted cows in week 1 and declined further to 26.4 ± 0.8 kg/d in week 3 of period 2 (Figure 4). Within the same time, milk production in the control group declined from 32.8 ± 0.8 kg/d (week 0) to 29.5 ± 1.1 kg/d (week 3 of period 2) as lactation curve decreased. Despite the high induced NEB, restricted cows showed only a moderate, though significantly reduced milk yield (27.4 ± 0.5 kg/d on average) during the three weeks of feed-restriction compared to C-cows (30.5 ± 0.7 kg/d; $P < 0.05$). The reduction in the present study of ~ 10% compared to the C-cows was less compared to the reduction of about 20% in milk yield in studies with a comparable extent of the induced NEB to the present study (Velez and Donkin, 2005; Carlson et al., 2006). Among the level of the NEB induced by feed-restriction, its initiation and duration must be considered. In the present study, feed-restriction lasted for 3 weeks starting at 100 DIM, whereas feed restriction lasted only 5 days in the study of Carlson et al. (2006), but began at 132 DIM. Furthermore, parity (primiparous or multiparous), breed type, and also genetic merit of the dairy cow may influence a cow's adaptive response to a deliberately induced NEB. During the realimentation period, milk yield increased up to 29.6 ± 1.1 kg/d in restricted cows and declined thereafter similarly as in the control group with proceeding lactation (Figure 4). Milk yield in restricted cows fully recovered to the level of control cows, which can be attributed to the ad libitum feeding in the realimentation period. Contrary to the present results, milk yield of feed-restricted dairy cows in the study of Röhrmoser and Kirchgessner (1982) did not completely recover. In their study, ad libitum intake of feed was calculated to meet energy requirements of the control group. However, feed-restricted cows did not fully increase milk yield, but partly replenished body reserves that were mobilized previously.

Milk solubles and the milk fat-protein-ratio

Besides milk yield, milk composition was affected by lactational stage and energy status in the present study. Milk fat content was highest in week 1 p.p. (5.48 ± 0.12%), declined to 4.00 ± 0.08% in week 7 p.p. and increased slightly thereafter (Figure 7).

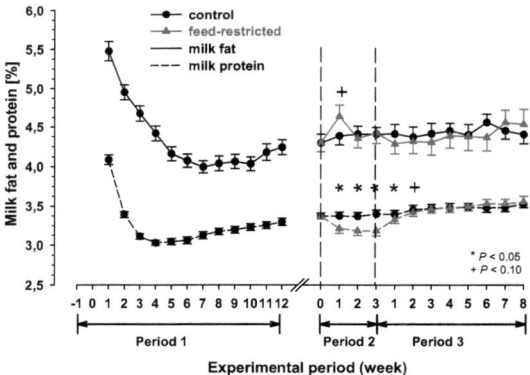

Figure 7. Milk fat and protein content (%) in cows during the experimental periods. Differences between the groups in period 2 and 3 are indicated with + ($P < 0.10$) and * ($P < 0.05$).

In week 0 of period 2, milk fat content averaged 4.30 ± 0.11%. Only in the first week of feed-restriction, there was a tendency for higher milk fat percentage in R-cows ($P < 0.10$) than in C-cows (4.63 ± 0.15% and 4.38 ± 0.11%, respectively). During the rest of period 2 and the following realimentation period, no differences were found between the two groups, supporting Velez and Donkin (2005) and Carlson et al. (2006) despite a comparable NEB induced by feed-restriction. Milk fat content multiplied with milk yield results in the average fat yield secreted by milk (Figure 8). Milk fat yield increased from week 1 p.p. (1,506 ± 52 g/d) to a maximum in week 3 p.p. (1,712 ± 53 g/d) and decreased thereafter to 1,419 ± 45 g/d in week 12 p.p. (Figure 8). At the initiation of energy-restriction (week 0 of period 2), daily milk fat yield was 1,384 ± 30 g/d over all cows. Over the entire restriction period, milk fat yield was lower for R-cows compared with C-cows (1,211 ± 22 vs. 1,335 ± 29 g/d; $P < 0.05$). During realimentation in period 3, milk fat yield decreased with decreasing milk yield in both groups until the end of the study (Figure 8).

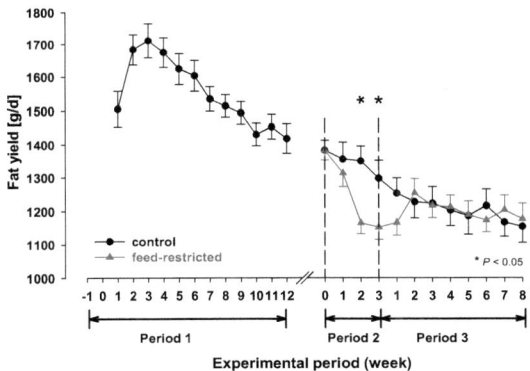

Figure 8. Milk fat yield (g/d) in cows during the experimental periods. Differences between the groups in period 2 and 3 are indicated with * ($P < 0.05$).

Similarly to milk fat content, milk protein content was highest in week 1 p.p. (4.09 ± 0.06%), declined to a nadir in week 4 p.p. (3.03 ± 0.04%) and increased thereafter to 3.30 ± 0.05% in week 12 p.p. (Figure 7). In period 2, milk protein concentration in R-cows was lower ($P < 0.05$) than in C-cows (3.19 ± 0.03% and 3.38 ± 0.03%, respectively), and the mean daily protein yield (Figure 9; calculated by multiplying milk yield with milk protein content) over the entire restriction period was lower in R-cows during period 2 (868 ± 13 vs. 1,027 ± 22 g/d; $P < 0.05$). The decrease in milk protein during the feed-restriction in period 2 can be attributed to the energy deficiency and the simultaneous reduced protein supply. These results

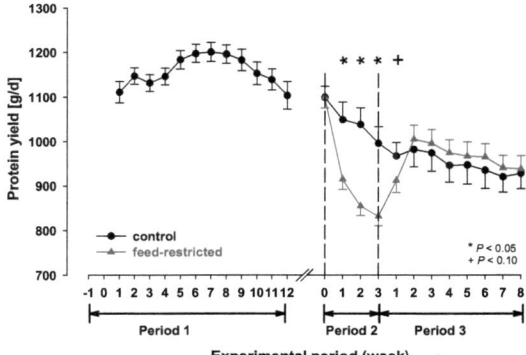

Figure 9. Milk protein yield (g/d) in cows during the experimental periods. Differences between the groups in period 2 and 3 are indicated with + ($P < 0.10$) and * ($P < 0.05$).

support studies of Röhrmoser and Kirchgessner (1982) and Carlson et al. (2006), and reflect the decreased ACP-balance during feed-restriction (Figure 6). During realimentation (period 3), R-cows had still a lower milk protein content compared to C-cows ($P < 0.05$), and in week 2 of period 3, there was still a tendency ($P < 0.10$) for lower protein percentage in the restricted cows (Figure 7).

As milk fat and milk protein content changed with altering energy status in dairy cows, out of these milk constituents the milk fat-protein-ratio was calculated to indicate a NEB.

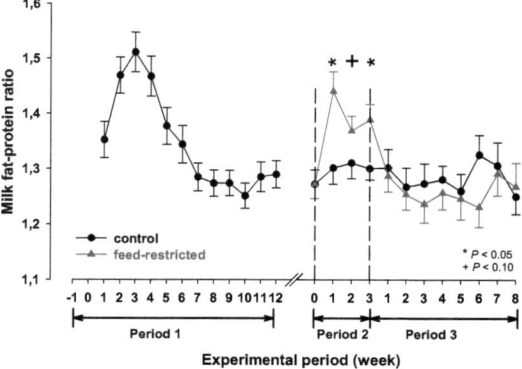

Figure 10. Milk fat-protein ratio in cows during the experimental periods. Differences between the groups in period 2 and 3 are indicated with + ($P < 0.10$) and * ($P < 0.05$).

The fat-protein-ratio increased from 1.35 ± 0.03 in week 1 p.p. to a maximum of 1.51 ± 0.04 in week 3 p.p. and declined to relatively constant values around 1.3 from week 7 to 12 p.p. (Figure 10). In week 0 of feed-restriction, the milk fat-protein-ratio averaged 1.27 ± 0.03 (Figure 10). Within one week of restriction, the fat-protein-ratio increased to 1.44 ± 0.04 and declined slightly thereafter (Figure 10). In period 3 (realimentation), the fat-protein-ratio stayed at the level of around 1.3 and did not differ anymore between the two groups. Heuer et al. (1999) recommend threshold values between 1.35 and 1.50 beyond which individual cows are regarded at higher risk for energy deficiency. Restricted cows showed a higher mean fat-protein-ratio than the control group in period 2 (1.40 ± 0.03 vs. 1.30 ± 0.03; $P < 0.05$). When 1.35 was considered as lower threshold, dairy cows in the present study were above this level during week 1 to 5 p.p. and during the entire feed-restriction period (Figure 10). However, it must be considered that in cases of rumen acidosis milk fat content might be depressed. Thus, the milk fat-protein-ratio would not indicate a NEB during rumen acidosis. In the present study, the facilitation of rumen acidosis was prevented by slowly increasing supply with concentrate. Therefore, the fat-protein-ratio in milk seems to be a suitable instrument to detect a NEB in early and mid lactation.

Milk lactose content increased rapidly from 4.46 ± 0.02% in week 1 p.p. to relatively constant values between 4.70 and 4.80% in week 3 p.p. onwards (Figure 11). Lactose content in milk was not affected by feed-restriction in the present study. In earlier studies of Velez and Donkin (2005) and Carlson et al. (2006), who induced a NEB of comparable extent to the present study, milk lactose was neither affected by feed-restriction.

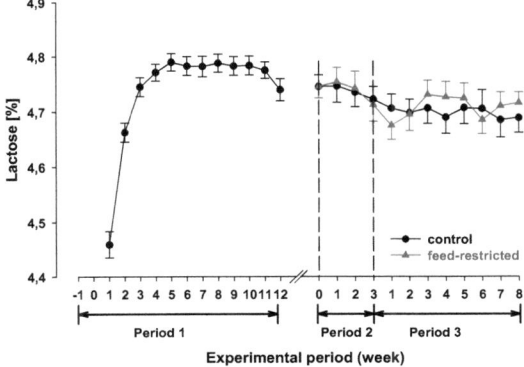

Figure 11. Milk lactose content (%) in cows during the experimental periods.

Body weight and body condition parameters

The mobilization of body reserves in dairy cows – mainly fat stores and to some extent proteins – enables the adaptation to energy and nutrient deficiencies. Mean BW declined from 715 ± 9 kg in week 1 a.p. to 668 ± 9 kg in week 1 p.p. (Figure 12). Due to the mobilization of body reserves, BW declined further to 647 ± 8 kg in week 4 p.p. and remained ~ 650 kg from week 7 to 12 p.p. in the present study (Figure 12).

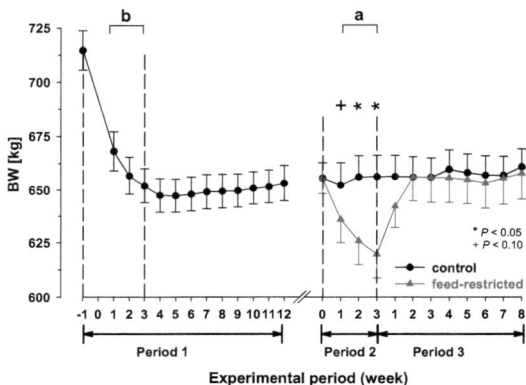

Figure 12. Body weight (BW; kg) of cows during the experimental periods. Differences between the groups in period 2 and 3 are indicated with + ($P < 0.10$) and * ($P < 0.05$). Differences between period 1 (week 1 to 3 p.p.) and period 2 are indicated with different letters (a,b; $P < 0.05$).

At the initiation of feed-restriction, BW averaged 656 ± 7 kg over all cows. Within the first week of restriction, BW declined to 636 ± 11 kg and further to 620 ± 11 kg in week 3 of period 2 for R-cows. During feed-restriction in week 2 and 3, BW was lower for R-cows compared to C-cows ($P < 0.05$). BW of control-fed cows was constantly ~ 655 kg during periods 2 and 3 (Figure 12). During feed-restriction, the loss of BW is a consequence of the reduced DMI and the loss of gut fill (NRC, 2001). Yet, the amount of mobilized fat can be larger than the loss of BW, as depleted body mass was partially replaced by water in the tissues (Schröder and Staufenbiel, 2006). The mean decline of BW during the first 3 weeks p.p. compared to week 1 a.p. was higher than the decline of BW during the three weeks of feed-restriction (56 ± 4 kg vs. 23 ± 3 kg; $P < 0.05$). However, the weight of the foetus is included in cows` BW ante partum. The decline of BW after parturition during the NEB was comparable to the decline during feed-restriction in period 2. After the deliberately induced

NEB, BW in restricted cows recovered totally within 2 weeks of realimentation (Figure 12). Within the first week of period 3, BW increased from 620 ± 11 kg up to 642 ± 10 kg in R-cows. The positive energy balance for R-cows in realimentation, however, allowed only a replenishment of ~ 400g/d of body reserves. The quick increase of BW may therefore be attributed to the increased gut fill during the refeeding period and not only to the recovery of body reserves.

In order to quantify the actual changes in body reserves during periods of a NEB, BCS, MD and BFT were evaluated in the present study. The BCS can mirror the nutritional status in dairy cows as it reflects changes in the subcutaneous fat layer, but BCS is influenced by subjective factors (Bruckmaier et al., 1998a). According to these authors, changes of the longissimus dorsi MD and BFT paralleled those of BCS and reflect alterations of whole-body fat content and muscle mass. Before parturition, cows had a BCS of 3.51 ± 0.05 in week 1 a.p. that declined 3.03 ± 0.04 in week 6 p.p. (Figure 13). Until week 12 p.p., BCS remained around 3.00. During feed-restriction, BCS declined to 2.76 ± 0.05 in week 3 of period 2 in R-cows, whereas C-cows showed a higher BCS of 3.05 ± 0.07 in week 3 of period 2 ($P < 0.05$). Cows responded in BCS to a NEB more intensely in week 1 to 3 p.p. (0.34 ± 0.04) than in period 2 (0.16 ± 0.03; $P < 0.05$). In the realimentation period, BCS increased again for restricted cows and did not differ from control cows.

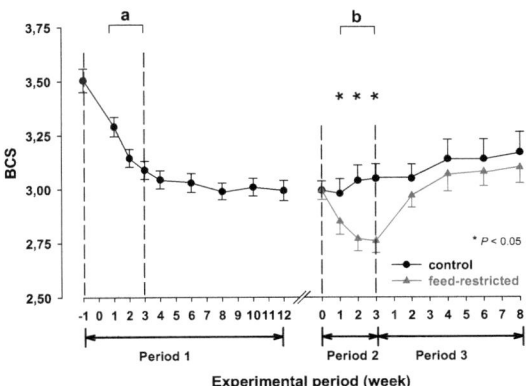

Figure 13. Body condition score (BCS) of cows during the experimental periods. Differences between the groups in period 2 and 3 are indicated with * ($P < 0.05$). Differences between period 1 (week 1 to 3 p.p.) and period 2 are indicated with different letters (a,b; $P < 0.05$).

BFT declined 4.6 ± 0.3 mm in week 1 a.p. to a nadir in week 10 p.p. (2.7 ± 0.2 mm; Figure 14). Within the first week of feed restriction, R-cows showed a rapid decline in BFT from 3.2 ± 0.2 mm to 2.2 ± 0.3 mm compared to C-cows, whose BFT increased to 3.3 ± 0.2 mm ($P < 0.05$). At the end of period 2, restricted cows had a lower BFT (3.7 ± 0.2 mm) than control cows (1.5 ± 0.2 mm; $P < 0.05$). The decrease of BFT during the restriction period was comparable to the mobilization in early lactation (0.8 ± 0.1 vs. 0.9 ± 0.1 mm). During realimentation (period 3), BFT in R-cows increased compared to C-cows, but did not recover during this period ($P < 0.05$; Figure 14).

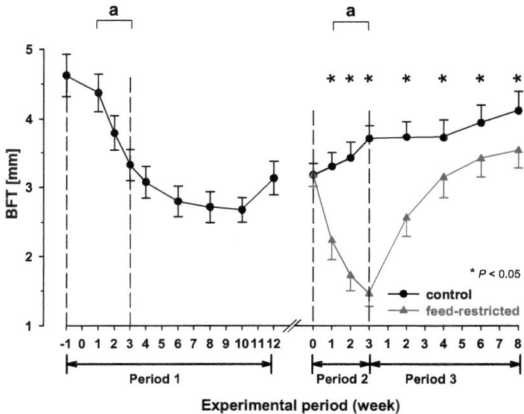

Figure 14. Backfat thickness (BFT; mm) of cows during the experimental periods. Differences between the groups in period 2 and 3 are indicated with * ($P < 0.05$). Differences between period 1 (week 1 to 3 p.p.) and period 2 are indicated with different letters (a,b; $P < 0.05$).

Similar to BFT, the decline of MD started in week 1 a.p. (45.5 ± 0.8 mm) until week 8 p.p. (38.1 ± 0.9 mm) and remained unchanged until week 12 p.p. (Figure 15). In period 2, MD of feed-restricted cows declined from initially 40.0 ± 0.8 mm to 36.1 ± 1.1 mm in week 3, whereas control cows had a higher MD of 40.3 ± 1.1 mm ($P < 0.05$). The decline of MD during the NEB in early lactation was higher compared to the decline during feed-restriction (3.5 ± 0.4 vs. 2.0 ± 0.4 mm; $P < 0.05$). In period 3, MD increased quickly for R-cows and was unchanged from week 4 onwards (Figure 15). MD recovered totally in the realimentation period, whereas BFT did not recover until the end of the experiment. Björntorp et al. (1982) showed that the replenishment of lipid stores after feed-restriction took longer than refilling protein stores. The priority of body protein is maintained by limited proteolysis via endocrine control during stages of a NEB (Hocquette et al., 2007).

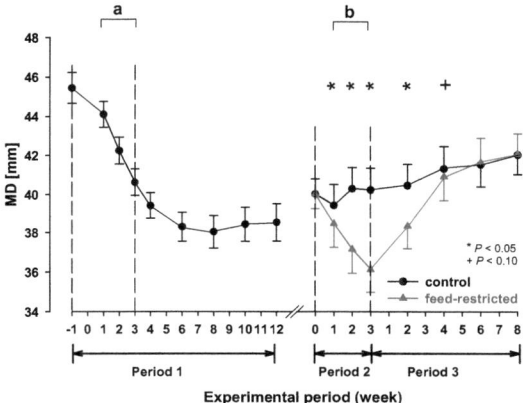

Figure 15. Muscle diameter (MD; mm) of the longissimus dorsi muscle in cows during the experimental periods. Differences between the groups in period 2 and 3 are indicated with + ($P < 0.10$) and * ($P < 0.05$). Differences between period 1 (week 1 to 3 p.p.) and period 2 are indicated with different letters (a,b; $P < 0.05$).

Animal Health

Homeorhesis does not guarantee overall metabolic equilibrium if the energy and nutrient resources are limited (Bruckmaier and van Dorland, 2010). The required metabolic adaptations can be successful but can also lead to metabolic disorders (Hachenberg et al., 2007; Kessel et al., 2008). A NEB can be responsible for health disorders, e.g., fertility problems or infectious diseases (Bertoni et al., 2009). On the other hand, health problems (e.g., digestive or locomotive problems) can be a trigger of a NEB and may affect the NEB negatively in early lactating cows. The incidence of disease occurrence is closely related to high yielding dairy cows in the transition period. A NEB represents a metabolic load, which has been defined as "the burden imposed by the synthesis and secretion of milk" (Knight et al., 1999). The present study shows that metabolically more stressed cows during the NEB in early lactation simultaneously have more health disorders compared to cows experiencing a higher deliberately induced NEB with lower responses in metabolism and also less health problems (Table 6). No differences were found between R- and C-group during feed-restriction ($P = 0.50$) and realimentation ($P = 0.35$; Table 6).

Table 6. Occurrence (quantity) of health disorders during experimental periods.

Health disorder	Period 1	Period 2			Period 3		
	R^1	R^1	C^2	P-value[3]	R^1	C^2	P-value
Mastitis and other udder related problems	8	-	2		4	1	
Reproductive tract related problems	2	-	-		-	-	
Claw problems	9	2	-		-	2	
Milk fever	3	-	-		-	-	
Total	**22**	**2**	**2**	**0.50**	**4**	**3**	**0.35**

[1] R: Feed-restricted cows
[2] C: Control cows
[3] P-values < 0.05 indicate significant differences between R- and C-cows

3.2 Adaptation of metabolites to a NEB

Blood glucose concentration

Glucose is an essential nutrient for milk lactose synthesis. Most of the glucose turnover, more than 80%, is used by the mammary gland for the synthesis of lactose during peak lactation (Bauman and Currie, 1980). Therefore, hepatic gluconeogenesis and glycogenolysis are increased to a maximum at the start of lactation. Despite these homeorhetic adaptations, a decrease of plasma glucose concentration after parturition is commonly observed. Glucose concentration was 4.01 ± 0.06 mmol/L in week 1 a.p. and dropped to a nadir of 3.30 ± 0.04 mmol/L in week 2 p.p. (Figure 16). According to previous studies (Baxter et al., 1956; Blum et al., 1983) this can be interpreted as a consequence of the high demand for this substrate, especially for the synthesis of lactose. Thereafter, glucose concentration increased up to 4.13 ± 0.07 mmol/L in week 12 p.p. (Figure 16). For control cows, plasma glucose increased slightly from 3.99 ± 0.04 mmol/L in week 0 of period 2 up to 4.15 ± 0.07 mmol/L in week 8 of period 3. Contrary, plasma glucose decreased significantly during the feed-restriction period in R-cows. Throughout period 2, mean plasma glucose concentrations were lower in feed-restricted cows than in control cows (3.85 vs. 4.06 mmol/L; $P < 0.05$), and increased again in period 3 to similar levels as C-cows (Figure 16). The decrease of plasma glucose concentration was greater during period 1 (0.65 ± 0.06 mmol/L) than in period 2 (0.16 ± 0.02 mmol/L; $P < 0.05$), despite the high induced NEB of almost 50% of requirements. Contrary to the findings of the present study, blood glucose concentration in mid lactation was not affected by a partial energy-restriction in the study of Carlson et al. (2006) despite a similar extent of the induced NEB.

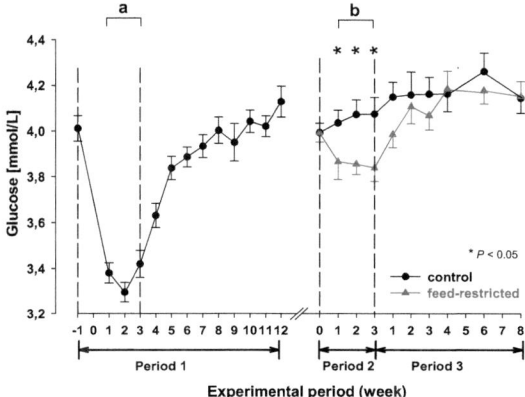

Figure 16. Plasma glucose concentration (mmol/L) in cows during the experimental periods. Differences between the groups in period 2 and 3 are indicated with * ($P < 0.05$). Differences between period 1 (week 1 to 3 p.p.) and period 2 are indicated with different letters (a,b; $P < 0.05$).

Blood NEFA concentration

As glucose is not available as energy source for dairy cows, body fat reserves become the main energy source during a NEB among volatile FA from the rumen. While mobilization of body reserves during the NEB in early lactation, nonesterified fatty acids (NEFA) are released from adipose tissue by lipolysis while lipogenesis is simultaneously reduced (Butler and Smith, 1989; Butler et al., 2003; Kessel et al., 2008). In week 1 a.p., plasma NEFA concentration averaged 0.23 ± 0.02 mmol/L (Figure 17). After parturition, NEFA concentrations in the present study increased up to week 2 p.p. (0.90 ± 0.06 mmol/L), then decreased until week 12 p.p. to 0.16 ± 0.01 mmol/L (Figure 17). In period 2, for R-cows, NEFA concentrations increased within the first week of feed-restriction from 0.13 ± 0.01 mmol/L to 0.27 ± 0.03 mmol/L, and gradually decreased thereafter. In period 3, plasma NEFA concentrations were similar for restricted cows and control cows ~ 0.10 mmol/L (Figure 17). The increase of plasma NEFA concentration was more intense in period 1 (0.59 ± 0.05 mmol/L) than in period 2 (0.08 ± 0.02 mmol/L; $P < 0.05$). For single cows in the present study, NEFA concentration increased up to 1.83 mmol/L in early lactation, whereas during the feed-restriction period a maximum of 0.80 mmol/L was reached. These findings are confirmed by Carlson et al. (2006), who found that plasma NEFA concentrations in feed-restricted cows (132 DIM) were elevated much less compared to the observations in early lactation. When the hepatic uptake of NEFA exceeds the capacity for oxidation and secretion

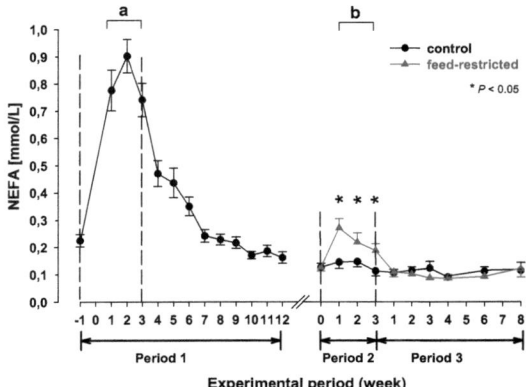

Figure 17. Plasma NEFA concentration (mmol/L) in cows during the experimental periods. Differences between the groups in period 2 and 3 are indicated with * ($P < 0.05$). Differences between period 1 (week 1 to 3 p.p.) and period 2 are indicated with different letters (a,b; $P < 0.05$).

of lipids via VLDL by the liver as observed during excessive mobilization of adipose tissue, NEFA are re-esterified and stored as triacylglycerol in the liver, which decreases metabolic functions of the liver and leads to fatty liver (Rukkwamsuk et al., 2000).

Blood BHBA concentration

As reported in van Knegsel (2007), the final common pathway for oxidation of NEFA and rumen derived volatile FA involves the oxidation of acetyl-CoA and oxaloacetate to form citrate. In a series of intermediate reactions of the Krebs cycle, citrate is metabolized to produce available ATP, NADH and $FADH_2$. NADH and $FADH_2$ can react with oxygen to produce ATP as energy source. During the NEB in early lactation, the production of acetyl-CoA from acetate, butyrate and NEFA released from body reserves is limited as at the same time oxaloacetate is needed for the synthesis of glucose. Consequently, the accumulated acetyl-CoA is directed to the formation of ketone bodies, i.e. acetone, BHBA and acetoacetate (Berg et al., 2006), which may cause ketosis. Ketone bodies may also originate from butyrate from ruminal fermentation and subsequent metabolization in the ruminal epithelium (Kristensen et al., 2000), but its concentration in blood, milk, and urine are closer linked to lipolysis than to ruminal absorption.

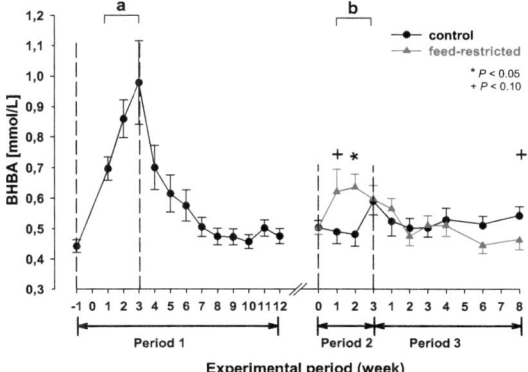

Figure 18. Plasma BHBA concentration (mmol/L) in cows during the experimental periods. Differences between the groups in period 2 and 3 are indicated with + ($P < 0.10$) and * ($P < 0.05$). Differences between period 1 (week 1 to 3 p.p.) and period 2 are indicated with different letters (a,b; $P < 0.05$).

In the present study, the concentration of BHBA increased from 0.44 ± 0.02 mmol/L in week 1 a.p. to a maximum of 0.98 ± 0.14 mmol/L in week 3 p.p. during the NEB in early lactation (Figure 18). These results support the findings of Doepel et al. (2002), who showed that plasma BHBA concentration peaked later than NEFA concentration. In the study of Kessel et al. (2008), a threshold of 1 mmol/L for BHBA was used to identify hyperketotic cows. On average this threshold was not exceeded in the present study, though plasma BHBA concentrations of single cows reached 2.25 mmol/L. Thereafter, BHBA decreased to a steady concentration ~ 0.50 mmol/L from week 7 to 12 p.p. (Figure 18). During feed-restriction in period 2, BHBA concentrations increased from 0.50 mmol/L to a peak of 0.64 mmol/L in R-cows in week 2 (Figure 18), where BHBA concentrations were higher compared to C-cows (0.48 ± 0.04 mmol/L; $P < 0.05$). For single cows, the BHBA concentration (1.01 mmol/L) during feed-restriction reached the threshold of 1 mmol/L given in Kessel et al. (2008). In period 1, cows responded with a greater increase (0.41 ± 0.07 mmol/L) in BHBA concentrations to a NEB than in period 2 (0.13 ± 0.03 mmol/L; $P < 0.05$). In period 3, BHBA concentrations of R-cows declined to the level of C-cows (Figure 18). In the study of Carlson et al. (2006), an energy-restriction of 50% did not increase BHBA concentration in feed-restricted cows. This can be explained by the smaller rise in the concentration of NEFA during the nutrition induced NEB that serve as a substrate for ketone body production. In general, plasma metabolites responded to the deliberately induced NEB at the same time as to the lactation NEB, but the extent of changes was lower.

3.3 Adaptations of endocrine and hepatic gene expression parameters to a NEB

Plasma insulin concentration, RQUICKI and gene expression of INSR

The endocrine system mediates essential signals for the successful implementation and maintenance of lactation. The state of hypoinsulinemia in early lactating dairy cows is a major regulatory element in the adaptive system around parturition to support lactation (Butler et al., 2003).

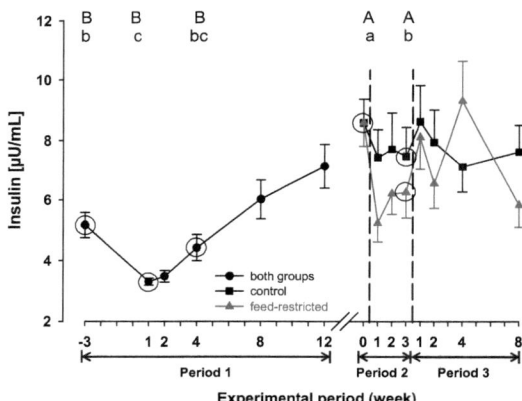

Figure 19. Plasma concentration of insulin (µU/mL) in cows during the experimental periods. Changes over time for points with simultaneous blood and liver samples (in circles) within the groups in period 1 (week 3 a.p., week 1 p.p., week 4 p.p.) and period 2 (week 0 and 3) are marked with different letters (A-B for the control group; a-c for the feed-restricted group; $P < 0.05$).

The decreased plasma insulin concentrations during the NEB in early lactation in the present study reduce glucose uptake in insulin-responsive tissues (e.g., muscle and adipose tissue) and enable more glucose uptake of the non-insulin-responsive mammary gland (Bauman and Elliot, 1983) via insulin-independent glucose transporters GLUT 1 and 3 (Zhao et al., 1996). Along with enhanced sensitivity to effects of catecholamines, the insulin resistance in early lactation is one of the main triggers to activate hormone-sensitive lipases in adipose tissue and hence fat mobilization. Furthermore, insulin is hypothesized to be a key signal regulating the coupling of the somatotropic axis (Butler et al., 2003).

Insulin concentration in period 1 decreased from week 3 a.p. (5.2 ± 0.4 µU/mL) to a minimum in week 1 p.p. (3.3 ± 0.1 µU/mL) and increased thereafter to 7.1 ± 0.7 µU/mL in week 12 p.p. (Figure 19). For restricted cows, insulin concentration was lower in week 3 of period 2 (6.2 ± 0.9 µU/mL) compared to week 0 of period 2 (8.6 ± 0.8 µU/mL; $P < 0.05$). During period 2, insulin concentration was not significantly different between the feed-restricted and the control group. Insulin concentration for R-cows was lower in week 1 p.p. (3.4 ± 0.5 µU/mL) compared to week 3 of period 2 (6.2 ± 0.9 µU/mL; $P < 0.05$). In period 3, no differences were detected for insulin between R- and C-group (Figure 19).

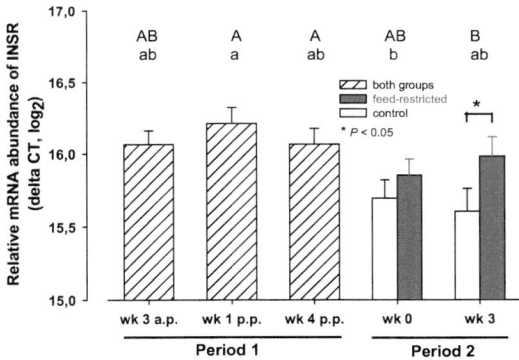

Figure 20. Relative liver mRNA abundance (delta CT, log$_2$) of insulin receptor (INSR) in cows over the time points. Effects of feed-restriction on mRNA abundance for cows during period 2 are marked with * ($P < 0.05$). Changes over time within the groups in period 1 (week 3 a.p., week 1 p.p., week 4 p.p.) and period 2 (week 0 and 3) are marked with different letters (A-B for the control group; a-b for the feed-restricted group; $P < 0.05$).

Expression of INSR in period 1 increased from week 3 a.p. to a maximum in week 1 p.p. and decreased thereafter (Figure 20). Between week 0 and week 3 of period 2, no differences were found in expression of INSR for R- and C-group. In week 3 of period 2, R-cows had a higher mRNA abundance of INSR compared to C-cows ($P < 0.05$). For R-cows, mRNA abundance of INSR between day 3 p.p. and week 3 of period 2 did not differ (Figure 20).

Due to feed-restriction, the deliberately induced NEB study was accompanied by a protein deficiency expressed by the ACP balance, which would explain the rather small decline in plasma insulin concentration compared to the decline in early lactation (Ronge et al., 1988;

Kreuzer et al., 1991). The mRNA abundance of hepatic INSR was highest during the NEB in early lactation and also in cows during the deliberately induced NEB. It appears that the low plasma insulin level causes an upregulation of the INSR, perhaps to maintain the insulin function in the liver while maximizing nutrient supply to the mammary gland.

In dairy cows selected for high milk production, peri- and post-parturient insulin resistance plays a pivotal role both in the adaptation to the NEB, and in the pathogenesis of some NEB-related diseases (Kerestes et al., 2009), such as excessive lipid accumulation in the liver (Ohtsuka et al., 2001; Grummer, 2008) and ketosis (Hove, 1978).

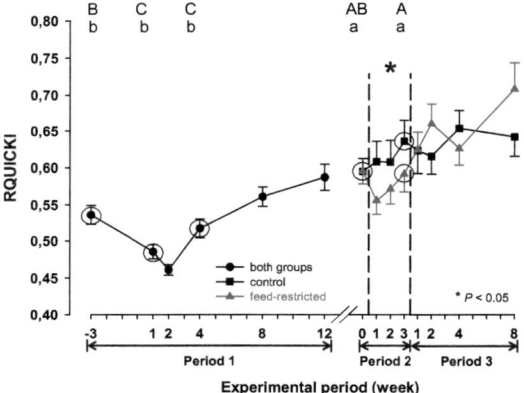

Figure 21. The revised quantitative insulin sensitivity check index (RQUICKI) in cows during the experimental periods. Differences between the groups in period 2 and 3 are indicated with * ($P < 0.05$). Changes over time for points with simultaneous blood and liver samples (in circles) within the groups in period 1 (week 3 a.p., week 1 p.p., week 4 p.p.) and period 2 (week 0 and 3) are marked with different letters (A-C for the control group; a-b for the feed-restricted group; $P < 0.05$).

The RQUICKI has been introduced by Holtenius and Holtenius (2007) to detect mild differences in insulin resistance in healthy, lactating dairy cows. In the study of Kerestes et al. (2009), however, the RQUICKI was not correlated with insulin resistance in dairy cows with ketosis or puerperal metritis. The present study showed a decrease of RQUICKI from 0.54 ± 0.01 in week 3 a.p. to a nadir of 0.46 ± 0.01 in week 2 p.p. (Figure 21) during NEB indicating insulin resistance during early lactation and thereby facilitating nutrient uptake by the mammary gland. RQUICKI remained almost unchanged during the deliberately induced NEB in later lactation and did not decrease that much as compared to early lactation, i.e. an insulin resistance did not occur during this period. Between week 0 and week 3 of period 2, RQUICKI of R- and C-cows did not differ (Figure 21). On average, RQUICKI was lower for R-cows compared to C-cows during period 2 (0.57 ± 0.02 vs. 0.62 ± 0.03; $P < 0.05$). Restricted cows had a lower RQUICKI during the NEB in week 1 p.p. compared to week 3 of period 2 ($P < 0.05$). In period 3, RQUICKI did not differ between groups. Stengärde et al. (2010) found the RQUICKI to be a more sensitive method for detection of metabolic imbalances than the individual parameters (NEFA, glucose, insulin) used for the calculation of the index. As genetically high yielding dairy cows show a higher insulin resistance than low yielding dairy cows (Chagas et al., 2009), the RQUICKI might also be related to differences in productivity.

Plasma GH, IGF-I and gene expression of GHR-1A, IGF-I and IGF-IR

GH and the other constituents of the somatotropic axis contribute markedly to adaptation processes in early lactation (Bauman and Currie, 1980; Bradford and Allen, 2008). Low circulating insulin is involved in the uncoupling of the somatotropic axis in the liver via down-regulation of the hepatic growth hormone receptor (Kobayashi et al., 1999; Rhoads et al., 2004). Consequently plasma GH levels increase, while plasma IGF-I concentrations remain low. A direct effect of GH is the stimulation of lipolysis from adipose tissue supported by enhanced sensitivity to β-adrenergic effects of catecholamines. While plasma insulin concentrations are low, the high levels of GH and NEFA induce an additional insulin resistance in the peripheral tissues (Bruckmaier and van Dorland, 2010).

The concentration of plasma GH increased from 4.87 ± 0.38 µg/L in week 3 a.p. to a maximum in week 1 p.p. (7.22 ± 0.60 µg/L) and then gradually decreased until week 12 p.p. (4.54 ± 0.28 µg/L; Figure 22). The increased GH secretion during the NEB p.p. enables the shift of nutrients from body stores towards the mammary gland for milk synthesis (Bauman et al., 1982). The plasma concentration of GH is increased around parturition, and remains elevated in early lactation (Bell, 1995; Block et al., 2001). Plasma GH concentration did not differ between week 0 and week 3 of period 2 in both groups. No differences in GH during feed-restriction and the following realimentation period were detected between the groups (Figure 21). The concentration of GH in the present study was greater during the NEB in early lactation than in the period following the NEB in agreement with Ronge et al. (1988) and Bradford and Allen (2008).

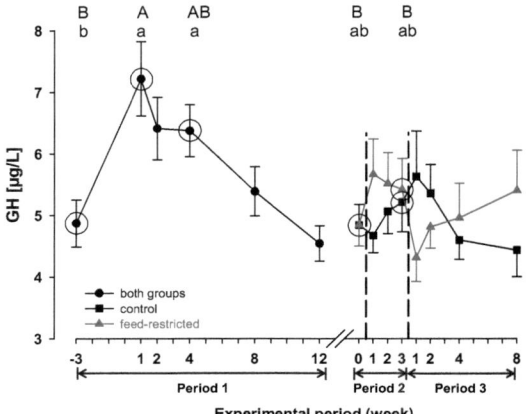

Figure 22. Plasma concentration of growth hormone (GH; µg/L) in cows during the experimental periods. Changes over time for points with simultaneous blood and liver samples (in circles) within the groups in period 1 (week 3 a.p., week 1 p.p., week 4 p.p.) and period 2 (week 0 and 3) are marked with different letters (A-B for the control group; a-b for the feed-restricted group; $P < 0.05$).

The GHR 1A transcript is found only in postnatal liver and accounts for ~ 50% of total hepatic GHR mRNA in well-fed prepartum dairy cows (Kobayashi et al., 1999; Lucy et al., 2001). Its abundance drops by > 50% at parturition, but recovers substantially over the first 2 weeks of lactation (Kobayashi et al., 1999; Radcliff et al., 2003). A decreased GHR 1A expression accounts for decreased GHR abundance, and therefore for reduced synthesis of IGF-I in periparturient dairy cows (Kim et al., 2004; Radcliff et al., 2003). Also the periparturient down-regulation of the hepatic GH receptor, and of hepatic IGF-I could be demonstrated at the mRNA level (Radcliff et al., 2003; Rhoads et al., 2008). Due to the lacking feedback via IGF-I, plasma GH concentrations increase, and exert mainly a direct lipolytic effect in adipose tissue. The present study showed the characteristic down-regulation of the mRNA abundance of GHR 1A during the NEB p.p., which is thought to be a key change during the uncoupling of the somatotropic axis in early lactation (Ronge et al., 1988; Lucy et al., 2001; McCarthy et al., 2009). The highest mRNA abundance of GHR 1A compared to the other time-points was measured for control cows in week 3 a.p. ($P < 0.05$), whereas restricted cows did not show a difference in gene expression over time (Figure 23). In period 2, there was no difference in mRNA abundance of GHR 1A between week 0 and week 3 for the groups. In week 3 of period 2, no differences in gene expression of GHR 1A were found between the feed-restricted and the control group.

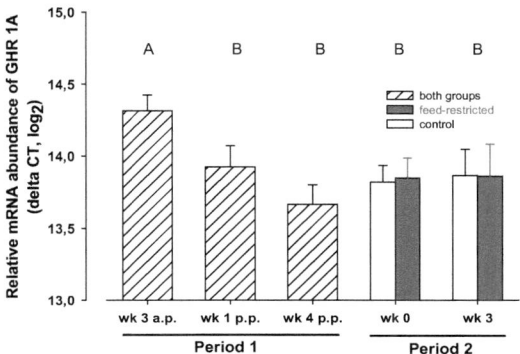

Figure 23. Relative liver mRNA abundance (delta CT, $\log_2$) of GH receptor 1A (GHR 1A) in cows over the time points. Changes over time within the groups in period 1 (week 3 a.p., week 1 p.p., week 4 p.p.) and period 2 (week 0 and 3) are marked with different letters (A-B for the control group; $P < 0.05$).

As a consequence of the uncoupling of the somatotropic axis, plasma IGF-I concentration decreased from 170.3 ± 7.4 ng/mL in week 3 a.p. to 65.6 ± 4.6 ng/mL in week 2 p.p. and increased to 108.3 ± 5.7 ng/mL in week 12 p.p. (Figure 24). Plasma IGF-I concentration did not differ between week 0 and week 3 of period 2 in both groups. IGF-I concentration was lower on average in the restricted group compared to the control group during period 2 (98.3 ± 8.2 vs. 111.7 ± 7.4 ng/mL; $P < 0.05$). In the realimentation period (period 3), plasma concentration of IGF-I increased in R-cows to similar values compared to the control group (Figure 24).

Early lactating dairy cows show a depressed plasma IGF-I concentration (Block et al., 2001; Kobayashi et al., 1999), and lose the ability to mount a robust GH-dependent increase in plasma IGF-I (Ronge and Blum, 1989; Vicini et al., 1991). The decrease of plasma IGF-I means also a loss of negative feedback of GH secretion and hence a lack of inhibition of GH release from the pituitary and provides the explanation of high GH plasma concentrations during catabolic stages (Radcliff et al., 2006). These changes reflect the expected differences of hepatic IGF-I synthesis (Kobayashi et al., 1999; Butler et al., 2003; Wook Kim et al., 2004). In week 3 a.p. (period 1), mRNA abundance of IGF-I was highest compared to week 1 and week 4 p.p. for both, C- and R-group (Figure 25). The expression of IGF-I did not differ between week 0 and week 3 of period 2 for both groups. In week 3 of period 2, R-cows had a higher mRNA abundance than C-cows ($P < 0.05$), which was also higher compared to week 1 p.p. in period 1 ($P < 0.05$).

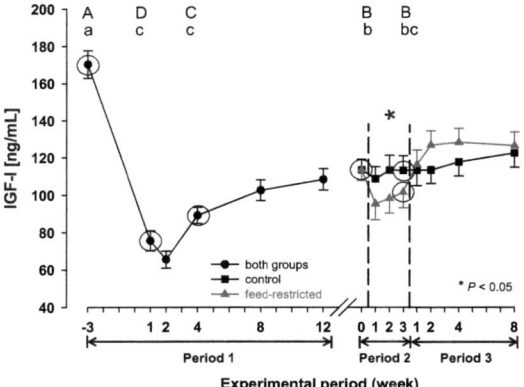

Figure 24. Plasma concentration of insulin-like growth factor-I (IGF-I; ng/mL) in cows during the experimental periods. Differences between the groups in period 2 and 3 are indicated with * ($P < 0.05$). Changes over time for points with simultaneous blood and liver samples (in circles) within the groups in period 1 (week 3 a.p., week 1 p.p., week 4 p.p.) and period 2 (week 0 and 3) are marked with different letters (A-D for the control group; a-c for the feed-restricted group; $P < 0.05$).

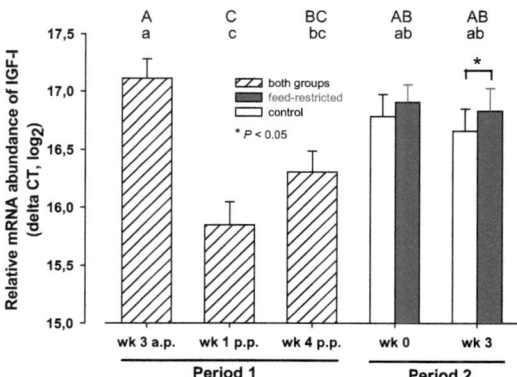

Figure 25. Relative liver mRNA abundance (delta CT, log$_2$) of IGF-I in cows over the time points. Effects of feed-restriction on mRNA abundance for cows during period 2 are marked with * ($P < 0.05$). Changes over time within the groups in period 1 (week 3 a.p., week 1 p.p., week 4 p.p.) and period 2 (week 0 and 3) are marked with different letters (A-C for the control group; a-c for the feed-restricted group; $P < 0.05$).

The mRNA abundance of IGF-IR was not affected over time within groups (Figure 26). Feed-restriction (week 3 in period 2) increased mRNA abundance of IGF-IR for R-cows compared to C-cows ($P < 0.05$). Gene expression of IGF-IR for R-cows did not differ during between the NEB in week 1 p.p. (period 1) and week 3 of period 2 (Figure 26).

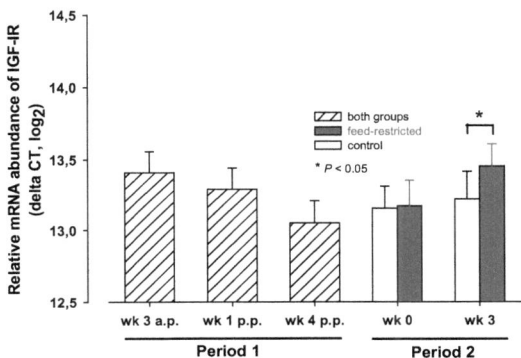

Figure 26. Relative liver mRNA abundance (delta CT, log$_2$) of IGF-I receptor (IGF-IR) in cows over the time points. Effects of feed-restriction on mRNA abundance for cows during period 2 are marked with * ($P < 0.05$).

The responses of plasma GH and IGF-I concentration to the deliberately induced NEB were similar directed to the NEB p.p., but the changes were less intense. In contrast to NEB in early lactation, feed-restriction did not decrease mRNA abundance of GHR 1A or of IGF-I indicating that the endocrine adaptation to the NEB is differently mediated in these two periods of NEB. Studies conducted later in lactation (153 to 265 DIM; Kobayashi et al., 2002) showed a decreased mRNA expression of hepatic IGF-I, but mRNA expression of GHR 1A was not changed. In a study with feed-restricted, but non-lactating dairy cows, decreased plasma IGF-I levels were observed during the period of induced NEB and occurred concomitantly with hepatic declining IGF-I mRNA and GHR 1A mRNA abundance (Meier et al., 2008). However, there was no increase in plasma GH level (Meier et al., 2008). These different findings illustrate a variety of different interactions between the key players of the somatotropic axis at different metabolic stages of dairy cows. The results of the present study indicate a partial uncoupling of the somatotropic axis during the deliberately induced NEB as the plasma IGF-I concentration and hepatic IGF-I mRNA abundance differed between the feed-restricted and control group while plasma GH was not different.

Gene expression of IGFBP-1, -2 and -3

The underlying partial GH resistance of the liver observed in the present study may be related to changes of IGFBPs to induce a mechanism for the preferential utilization of mobilized substrates to maintain homeostasis rather than cell growth and proliferation in the feed-restricted animals (Renaville et al., 2002). A higher mRNA abundance of IGFBP-1 and -2 was observed during the NEB in early lactation and deliberately induced NEB (Figures 27, 28). The mRNA abundance of IGFBP-1 in period 1 increased from week 3 a.p. to a maximum at week 1 p.p.. No differences were found for IGFBP-1 between week 0 and week 3 of period 2 for both, R- and C-group. R-cows showed a higher mRNA abundance of IGFBP-1 in week 3 of period 2 compared to C-cows ($P < 0.05$). Expression of IGFBP-1 for R-cows was higher in week 1 p.p. (period 1) compared to week 3 of period 2 ($P < 0.05$; Figure 27). IGFBP-1 gene transcription was shown to be elevated during reduced feed intake and its glucose counter-regulatory role (Baxter, 1993). Because the expression of IGFBP-1 has been shown to be suppressed by both insulin and IGF-I (Kelley et al., 1996) the low levels of these factors are most likely responsible for the elevated IGFBP-1 mRNA abundance during a NEB.

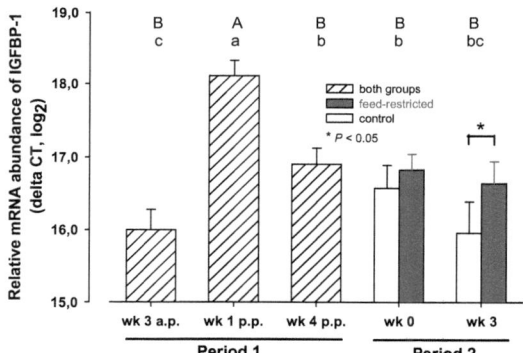

Figure 27. Relative liver mRNA abundance (delta CT, log$_2$) of IGF binding protein-1 (IGFBP-1) in cows over the time points. Effects of feed-restriction on mRNA abundance for cows during period 2 are marked with * ($P < 0.05$). Changes over time within the groups in period 1 (week 3 a.p., week 1 p.p., week 4 p.p.) and period 2 (week 0 and 3) are marked with different letters (A-B for the control group; a-c for the feed-restricted group; $P < 0.05$).

However, metabolic factors also may regulate IGFBP-2 in a manner similar to that of IGFBP-1. Low plasma insulin levels that occur during NEB trigger IGFBP-2 synthesis in the liver (Orlowski et al., 1990; Thissen et al., 1994). The mRNA abundance of IGFBP-2 in period 1 increased from week 3 a.p. to a maximum in week 1 p.p. for all cows and decreased until week 0 of period 2 (Figure 28). Neither R- nor C-group were different in expression of IGFBP-2 between week 0 and week 3 of period 2. In week 3 of period 2, R-cows had a higher expression of IGFBP-2 than C-cows ($P < 0.05$). IGFBP-2 was more upregulated in R-cows in week 1 p.p. (period 1) than in week 3 of period 2 ($P < 0.05$; Figure 28). The elevation of hepatic IGFBP-2 mRNA abundance during NEB in both lactational stages is consistent with the role of IGFBP to decrease the bioavailability of IGF-I for peripheral tissues (Vicini et al., 1991; Vandehaar et al., 1995; Fenwick et al., 2008).

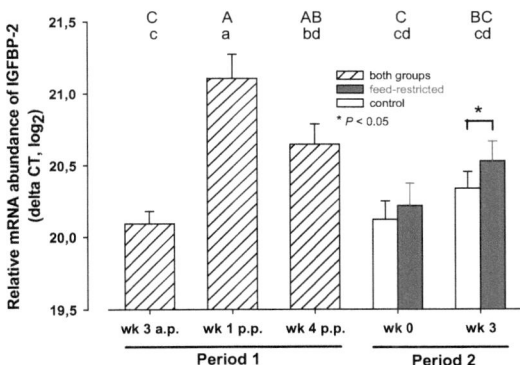

Figure 28. Relative liver mRNA abundance (delta CT, log$_2$) of IGFBP-2 in cows over the time points. Effects of feed-restriction on mRNA abundance for cows during period 2 are marked with * ($P < 0.05$). Changes over time within the groups in period 1 (week 3 a.p., week 1 p.p., week 4 p.p.) and period 2 (week 0 and 3) are marked with different letters (A-C for the control group; a-d for the feed-restricted group; $P < 0.05$).

The liver is the main contributor of IGFBP-3 in the circulation and GH is the main stimulator of IGFBP-3 (Kelley et al., 1996). In week 3 a.p., the mRNA abundance of IGFBP-3 was highest (Figure 29). Feed-restricted cows had a higher mRNA abundance of IGFBP-3 in week 3 of period 2 compared to control cows ($P < 0.05$). For R-cows, no differences were found in the expression of IGFBP-3 during the NEB between week 1 p.p. and week 3 of period 2. Whereas the mRNA of IGFBP-3 expression was decreased during the NEB in early lactation, feed-restricted cows in the present study showed a higher mRNA abundance of IGFBP-3 during the deliberately induced NEB compared to control cows (Figure 29). This demonstrates a difference between periods 1 and 2 in the adaptive response to NEB. Changes in IGFBP-1 and -2 during feed-restriction appear to restrict the insulin-like activity of IGF-I during catabolic states, but the major reduction of IGFBP-3 likely maximizes the availability of remaining IGF-I to the tissues (Breier, 1999). According to Breier (1999), circulating IGFBP-3 and its ternary complex are reduced during periods of NEB, and the activity of an IGFBP-3 specific protease is induced to reduce IGFBP-3 affinity for IGF-I. However, during the deliberately induced NEB in the present study the expression of IGFBP-3 did not change when compared to the beginning of feed-restriction. Despite decreased circulating IGF-I in feed-restricted cows, intact ternary complexes of IGF-I and IGFBP-3 appear to be changing that may alter the interpretation of action.

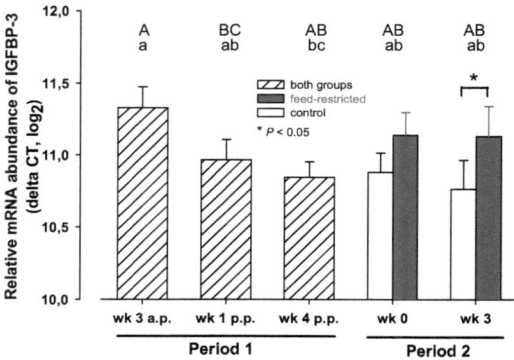

Figure 29. Relative liver mRNA abundance (delta CT, log$_2$) of IGFBP-3 in cows over the time points. Effects of feed-restriction on mRNA abundance for cows during period 2 are marked with * ($P < 0.05$). Changes over time within the groups in period 1 (week 3 a.p., week 1 p.p., week 4 p.p.) and period 2 (week 0 and 3) are marked with different letters (A-C for the control group; a-c for the feed-restricted group; $P < 0.05$).

Plasma concentration of leptin

Plasma leptin was shown to be positively regulated by fatness and to a lesser extent by the plane of nutrition in non-lactating sheep and cattle (Delavaud et al., 2002; Block et al., 2003b; Boisclair et al., 2006). Similar findings were reported for dairy cows, where the effects of adiposity appear attenuated during lactation (Block et al., 2003a; Liefers et al., 2003; Boisclair et al., 2006). A number of studies focused plasma leptin in high yielding dairy cows during the transition from pregnancy to lactation. In the present study, leptin concentration in plasma was highest during period 1 in week 3 a.p. (4.73 ± 0.20 ng/mL), reached a nadir in week 1 p.p. (3.38 ± 0.13 ng/mL), and thereafter increased gradually to 4.30 ± 0.21 ng/mL in week 12 p.p. (Figure 30). These results are confirmed by earlier studies (e.g., Block et al., 2001;

Liefers et al., 2003; Reist et al., 2003), who found that plasma concentration of leptin is highest during pregnancy and is reduced by 25-50% within a few days after parturition. Plasma leptin in the present study did not differ between week 0 and week 3 of period 2 for R-cows. Leptin was decreased significantly from 4.38 ± 0.19 ng/mL (week 0 in period 2) to 3.93 ± 0.22 ng/mL in restricted cows during feed-restriction compared to control cows (4.57 ± 0.29 ng/mL; $P < 0.05$). In period 3, no significant differences between the two groups were found (Figure 30).

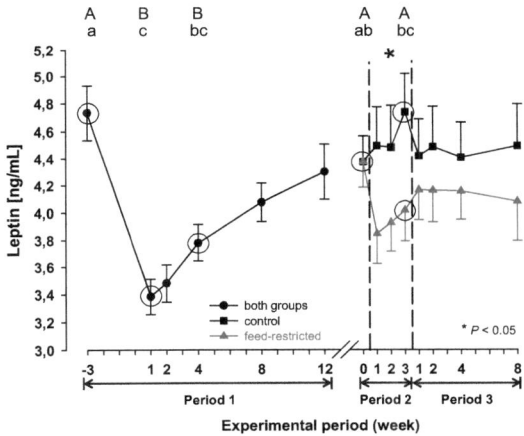

Figure 30. Plasma concentration of leptin (ng/mL) in cows during the experimental periods. Differences between the groups in period 2 and 3 are indicated * ($P < 0.05$). Changes over time for points with simultaneous blood and liver samples (in circles) within the groups in period 1 (week 3 a.p., week 1 p.p., week 4 p.p.) and period 2 (week 0 and 3) are marked with different letters (A-B for the control group; a-c for the feed-restricted group; $P < 0.05$).

In the present study, plasma leptin decreased in early lactating dairy cows as well as in feed-restricted cows. Block et al. (2001) attributed the reduction p.p. in plasma leptin to the state of NEB caused by the initiation of lactation associated with a reduced leptin gene expression in adipose tissue. Increased concentration of GH and decreased plasma insulin concentration coincide with the onset of NEB and the decline in plasma leptin in periparturient and underfed cows (Block et al., 2001; Block et al., 2003a). These observations suggested that reduced plasma leptin could represent decreased stimulation by insulin. The increased plasma GH of early lactation could also be involved in the fall of plasma leptin given its ability to antagonize insulin actions in adipose tissue (Bauman, 2000; Etherton and Bauman, 1998). It seems that increased β-adrenergic responsiveness of adipose tissue in early lactation also contributes to reduced leptin synthesis (Chilliard et al., 2001). Furthermore, leptin is partly responsible for maintaining T_4 levels (Vernon et al., 2002) and therefore hypoleptinemia may have been partially responsible for the hypothyroid state during periods of a NEB.

Plasma concentration of T_3, T_4 and the $T_3:T_4$-ratio

In period 1, plasma concentration of T_3 steadily increased from week 3 a.p. (0.82 ± 0.04 nmol/L) up to 1.29 ± 0.06 nmol/L in week 12 p.p. (Figure 31). Though the concentration of T_3 decreased on average in restricted cows compared to the control group during period 2 (1.18 ± 0.08 vs. 1.34 ± 0.07 nmol/L), changes were not significant. In the realimentation period, no differences were found between R- and C-group (Figure 31).

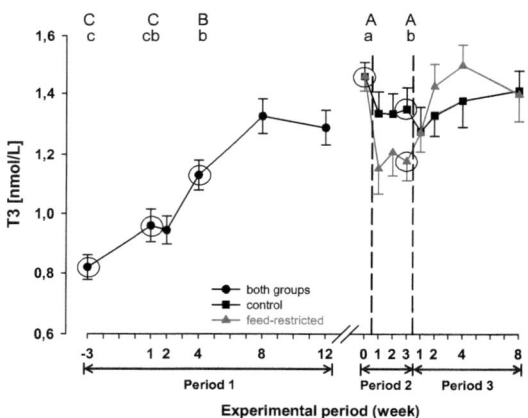

Figure 31. Plasma concentration of 3,5,3'-trijodthyronine (T_3; nmol/L) in cows during the experimental periods. Changes over time for points with simultaneous blood and liver samples (in circles) within the groups in period 1 (week 3 a.p., week 1 p.p., week 4 p.p.) and period 2 (week 0 and 3) are marked with different letters (A-C for the control group; a-c for the feed-restricted group; $P < 0.05$).

Contrary to T_3, plasma concentration of T_4 decreased from week 3 a.p. (64.5 ± 2.1 nmol/L) to a minimum in week 1 p.p. (41.7 ± 1.7 nmol/L) and increased thereafter up to 64.6 ± 2.7 nmol/L in week 12 p.p. (Figure 32). The concentration of T_4 did not significantly change between R- and C-group during feed-restriction (period 2) and remained unchanged in the realimentation period.

In period 1, the ratio of $T_3:T_4$ increased from the minimum in week 3 a.p. until week 1 p.p. and decreased slightly thereafter (Figure 33). In period 2, the $T_3:T_4$-ratio did not differ between the restricted and the control group. In period 3, no differences were found for the T_3:T_4-ratio between the groups. The effect of the deliberately induced NEB on thyroid hormones was less pronounced when compared to the NEB in early lactation. The results in agree with previous reports (Ronge et al., 1988; Pezzi et al., 2003). The results of the present study on changes in thyroid hormones during the induced NEB were confirmed by the findings of Windisch et al. (1991). Thyroid gland production of T_4 is normally transformed into T_3 by 5`-deiodination in the liver, but the deiodinating system is also present in other peripheral tissues that produce $T_3$ according to the local requirements (Pezzi et al., 2003). The increased utilization of thyroid hormones by the mammary gland or the altered 5`-deiodinase activity in liver are partly responsible for the hypothyroid state in early lactating animals. The hypothyroid state enhances mammary type II 5`-deiodinase and inhibits liver type I 5`-deiodinase activity (Pezzi et al., 2003). Therefore, a changed local T_3 production in the mammary gland might also be an important factor for reduced milk production during the NEB induced by feed-restriction.

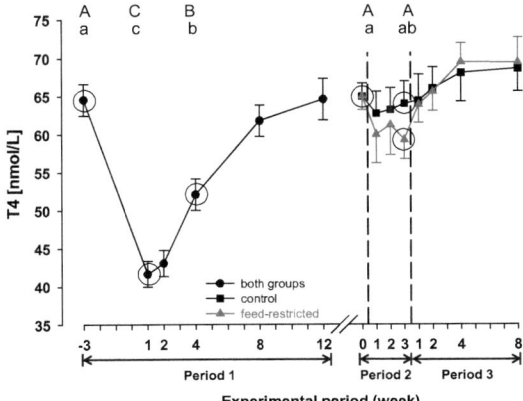

Figure 32. Plasma concentration of thyroxine (T_4; nmol/L) in cows during the experimental periods. Changes over time for points with simultaneous blood and liver samples (in circles) within the groups in period 1 (week 3 a.p., week 1 p.p., week 4 p.p.) and period 2 (week 0 and 3) are marked with different letters (A-C for the control group; a-c for the feed-restricted group; $P < 0.05$).

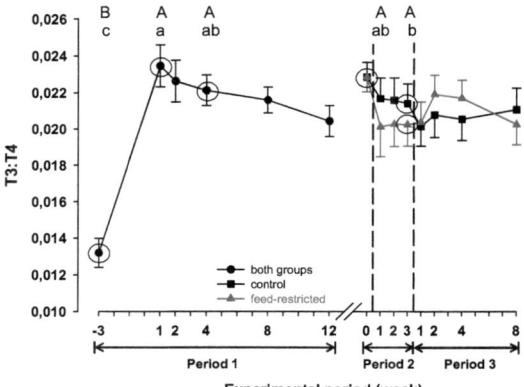

Figure 33. Ratio of $T_3:T_4$ in cows during the experimental periods. Changes over time for points with simultaneous blood and liver samples (in circles) within the groups in period 1 (week 3 a.p., week 1 p.p., week 4 p.p.) and period 2 (week 0 and 3) are marked with different letters (A-B for the control group; a-c for the feed-restricted group; $P < 0.05$).

3.4 Milk fatty acids and their relation to energy status

Changes in milk FA profile with altering energy status post partum

Milk fat content mainly determines energy requirements for milk production in dairy cows. Up to 98% of milk fat consists of triglycerides formed by glycerol and three fatty acids (FA) (Moate et al., 2007). Basically, milk fatty acids originate from four major pathways: the diet, the mammary gland (de novo synthesis), the rumen (biohydrogenation and bacterial degradation), and body fat mobilization (Stoop et al., 2009). Changes in milk FA composition during lactation originate from altered activities in these pathways (Van Knegsel et al., 2005; Stoop et al., 2009).

For the evaluation of changes in milk FA profile depending on a constant feeding regimen with continuous lactation, which reflects an altering energy status p.p., data from 30 dairy cows in period 1 and 20 cows of the control group in period 2 and 3 were investigated. Data on the energy status defined by energy balance, feed intake, milk yield and milk composition are given in chapter 3.1. The milk FA profile of cows with altering energy status p.p. in the present study is shown in table 7. With progressing lactation p.p. and improvement of energy balance through increasing feed intake, milk FA profile markedly changed. In the present study, most changes in milk FA profile took place during the observed NEB from week 1 to 6

Table 7. Changes in milk fatty acid (FA) composition in week 1, 4, 6, 12 (all animals), 17 and 21 (control group) post partum. Differences over time are marked with different superscripts ($P < 0.05$).

FA (g/100g FAME)	Week 1 (n=30)	Week 4 (n=30)	Week 6 (n=30)	Week 12 (n=30)	Week 17 (n=20)	Week 21 (n=20)
4:0	3.85^a ± 0.12	3.54^b ± 0.11	3.38^b ± 0.08	3.14^c ± 0.07	3.10^c ± 0.07	3.15^c ± 0.07
6:0	2.21^c ± 0.11	2.41^{ab} ± 0.08	2.55^a ± 0.05	2.40^{abc} ± 0.06	2.39^{abc} ± 0.04	2.34^{bc} ± 0.04
8:0	1.16^c ± 0.08	1.39^b ± 0.06	1.58^a ± 0.04	1.50^{ab} ± 0.04	1.51^{ab} ± 0.03	1.49^{ab} ± 0.02
10:0	2.24^c ± 0.18	2.82^b ± 0.16	3.52^a ± 0.13	3.52^a ± 0.10	3.61^a ± 0.08	3.56^a ± 0.06
10:1	0.12^d ± 0.01	0.21^c ± 0.01	0.27^b ± 0.01	0.31^{ab} ± 0.01	0.32^a ± 0.01	0.34^a ± 0.01
11:0	0.03^b ± 0.00	0.05^b ± 0.01	0.09^a ± 0.01	0.10^a ± 0.01	0.10^a ± 0.01	0.09^a ± 0.01
12:0	2.37^c ± 020	2.96^b ± 0.18	3.83^a ± 0.18	4.07^a ± 0.13	4.27^a ± 0.11	4.26^a ± 0.08
12:1	0.03^e ± 000	0.05^d ± 0.00	0.07^c ± 0.01	0.09^b ± 0.00	0.10^{ab} ± 0.00	0.10^a ± 0.00
13:0	0.07^c ± 0.00	0.09^c ± 0.01	0.14^b ± 0.01	0.15^{ab} ± 0.01	0.16^a ± 0.01	0.16^{ab} ± 0.01
14:0iso	0.07^b ± 0.00	0.06^b ± 0.01	0.07^b ± 0.01	0.08^b ± 0.01	0.10^a ± 0.00	0.11^a ± 0.01
14:0	8.82^c ± 0.48	9.75^b ± 0.32	11.36^a ± 0.28	12.06^a ± 0.23	12.18^a ± 0.17	12.22^a ± 0.14
14:1,9c	0.62^b ± 0.04	1.58^a ± 0.04	1.00^a ± 0.08	1.17^a ± 0.12	1.07^a ± 0.05	1.36^a ± 0.13
15:0iso	0.16^{cd} ± 0.01	0.15^d ± 0.01	0.17^c ± 0.00	0.20^b ± 0.01	0.22^a ± 0.01	0.23^a ± 0.00
15:0anteiso	0.27^d ± 0.01	0.31^c ± 0.01	0.38^b ± 0.02	0.42^a ± 0.01	0.44^a ± 0.01	0.45^a ± 0.01
15:0	0.64^c ± 0.03	0.74^c ± 0.05	0.98^b ± 0.09	1.15^{ab} ± 0.07	1.22^a ± 0.04	1.17^a ± 0.04
16:0iso	0.18^c ± 0.01	0.17^c ± 0.01	0.17^c ± 0.01	0.20^{bc} ± 0.01	0.22^{ab} ± 0.01	0.24^a ± 0.01
16:0	28.77^c ± 0.61	29.62^c ± 0.63	31.38^b ± 0.64	35.62^a ± 0.70	36.75^a ± 0.49	36.23^a ± 0.39
16:1,9c	2.31^a ± 0.16	2.27^a ± 0.14	1.93^b ± 0.12	1.84^b ± 0.08	1.78^b ± 0.06	1.82^b ± 0.05
17:0iso	0.19 ± 0.01	0.20 ± 0.02	0.21 ± 0.02	0.22 ± 0.02	0.19 ± 0.02	0.20 ± 0.02
17:0anteiso	0.36 ± 0.01	0.36 ± 0.01	0.35 ± 0.01	0.37 ± 0.02	0.36 ± 0.01	0.36 ± 0.01
17:0	0.46^a ± 0.01	0.38^b ± 0.02	0.37^b ± 0.02	0.38^b ± 0.02	0.36^b ± 0.01	0.34^b ± 0.01
17:1,9c	0.37^a ± 0.02	0.35^a ± 0.02	0.26^b ± 0.02	0.22^{bc} ± 0.02	0.19^c ± 0.01	0.19^c ± 0.01
18:0	12.88^a ± 0.33	10.87^b ± 0.29	10.17^b ± 0.36	8.92^c ± 0.28	8.56^c ± 0.22	8.54^c ± 0.17
18:1,9t	0.40 ± 0.03	0.39 ± 0.02	0.42 ± 0.01	0.42 ± 0.01	0.40 ± 0.01	0.42 ± 0.01
18:1,11t	1.01^{bc} ± 0.09	0.94^c ± 0.05	1.06^{bc} ± 0.04	1.11^{ab} ± 0.05	1.15^{ab} ± 0.04	1.23^a ± 0.04
18:1,9c	25.75^a ± 1.22	23.96^a ± 1.05	19.89^b ± 0.89	16.16^c ± 0.69	15.00^c ± 0.46	15.30^c ± 0.24

Table 7. (continued)

FA (g/100g FAME)	Week 1 (n=30)	Week 4 (n=30)	Week 6 (n=30)	Week 12 (n=30)	Week 17 (n=20)	Week 21 (n=20)
18:1,c11	1.06[a] ± 0.09	1.01[ab] ± 0.09	0.92[abc] ± 0.07	0.76[bcd] ± 0.08	0.68[cd] ± 0.06	0.63[d] ± 0.05
18:1,c12	0.24[c] ± 0.01	0.25[c] ± 0.01	0.26[bc] ± 0.01	0.26[bc] ± 0.01	0.29[ab] ± 0.01	0.29[a] ± 0.01
18:2,9c,12c	1.95 ± 0.05	1.89 ± 0.06	1.94 ± 0.06	1.84 ± 0.05	1.79 ± 0.04	1.77 ± 0.04
18:3,9c,12c,15c	0.38[ab] ± 0.01	0.34[bc] ± 0.01	0.35[bc] ± 0.01	0.33[c] ± 0.01	0.40[a] ± 0.01	0.39[a] ± 0.01
18:2,9c,11t	0.35[b] ± 0.02	0.34[b] ± 0.02	0.34[b] ± 0.01	0.37[b] ± 0.01	0.43[a] ± 0.01	0.48[a] ± 0.02
18:2,10t,12c	0.04 ± 0.01	0.03 ± 0.01	0.03 ± 0.01	0.02 ± 0.01	0.03 ± 0.01	0.03 ± 0.01
20:0	0.10 ± 0.01	0.09 ± 0.01	0.09 ± 0.01	0.10 ± 0.01	0.10 ± 0.00	0.10 ± 0.00
20:1,11c	0.06[a] ± 0.00	0.06[ab] ± 0.00	0.05[b] ± 0.00	0.04[c] ± 0.00	0.04[c] ± 0.00	0.03[c] ± 0.00
20:2,11c,14c	0.03[ab] ± 0.00	0.03[b] ± 0.00	0.03[a] ± 0.00	0.03[a] ± 0.00	0.03[a] ± 0.00	0.03[a] ± 0.00
21:0	0.02 ± 0.01	0.03 ± 0.01	0.03 ± 0.01	0.03 ± 0.01	0.03 ± 0.01	0.04 ± 0.01
20:3,8c,11c,14c	0.12[a] ± 0.01	0.09[b] ± 0.01	0.11[ab] ± 0.01	0.13[a] ± 0.01	0.14[a] ± 0.01	0.14[a] ± 0.01
20:4,5c,8c,11c,14c	0.17[a] ± 0.02	0.11[b] ± 0.01	0.11[b] ± 0.01	0.13[b] ± 0.01	0.12[b] ± 0.01	0.12[b] ± 0.01
20:5,5c,8c,11c,14c,17c	0.05[a] ± 0.00	0.04[b] ± 0.00	0.04[b] ± 0.00	0.04[ab] ± 0.00	0.04[ab] ± 0.00	0.04[ab] ± 0.00
22:0	0.04[b] ± 0.00	0.04[ab] ± 0.00	0.04[ab] ± 0.00	0.05[ab] ± 0.00	0.05[ab] ± 0.00	0.05[a] ± 0.00
22:5,7c,10c,13c,16c,19c	0.06 ± 0.01	0.05 ± 0.01	0.05 ± 0.01	0.06 ± 0.01	0.06 ± 0.01	0.07 ± 0.01
Summarized FA						
n6 FA	2.28[a] ± 0.06	2.13[ab] ± 0.06	2.20[ab] ± 0.06	2.13[ab] ± 0.06	2.09[b] ± 0.04	2.04[b] ± 0.05
n3 FA	0.49[ab] ± 0.02	0.43[c] ± 0.02	0.44[bc] ± 0.01	0.43[c] ± 0.02	0.51[a] ± 0.02	0.50[ab] ± 0.02
n6:n3-ratio	4.74[ab] ± 0.17	5.02[a] ± 0.16	5.04[a] ± 0.18	5.12[a] ± 0.22	4.28[b] ± 0.19	4.26[b] ± 0.14
CLA	0.38[b] ± 0.02	0.37[b] ± 0.02	0.37[b] ± 0.02	0.39[b] ± 0.02	0.46[a] ± 0.01	0.51[a] ± 0.02
trans FA	1.41[bc] ± 0.12	1.32[c] ± 0.07	1.48[abc] ± 0.05	1.53[ab] ± 0.05	1.55[ab] ± 0.04	1.65[a] ± 0.04
de novo syn. FA	22.63[c] ± 1.10	26.10[b] ± 1.06	29.38[a] ± 0.72	30.35[a] ± 0.61	30.80[a] ± 0.42	30.89[a] ± 0.33
total C16 FA	31.25[c] ± 0.59	32.06[bc] ± 0.63	33.48[b] ± 0.63	37.67[a] ± 0.72	38.76[a] ± 0.50	38.30[a] ± 0.41
preformed FA	46.11[a] ± 1.39	41.84[b] ± 1.23	37.14[c] ± 1.18	31.99[d] ± 1.01	30.44[d] ± 0.65	30.80[d] ± 0.39

post partum, while FA composition was relatively constant between week 12 to 21 p.p. (Table 7). Fatty acids up to C16:0 showed lowest proportions in week 1 p.p. that increased to relatively constant proportions in week 6 and 12, respectively, onwards (Table 7). These findings agree with earlier studies (Stull et al., 1966; Palmquist et al., 1993; Kay et al., 2005; Garnsworthy et al., 2006). The proportion of saturated fatty acids (SFA), especially C16:0 increased from week 1 (28.8 ± 0.6 g/100g FAME) to 12 p.p. (35.6 ± 0.7 g/100g FAME) in the present study (Figure 34), while monounsaturated fatty acids (MUFA), predominantly C18:1,9c decreased from 25.75 ± 1.22 g/100g FAME (week 1 p.p.) until week 12 p.p. (16.2 ± 0.7 g/100g FAME) with improving energy balance (Table 7).

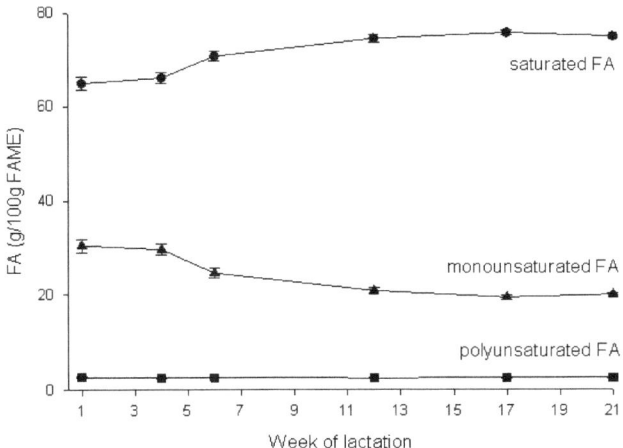

Figure 34. Changes in saturated FA (circles), monounsaturated FA (triangles) and polyunsaturated FA (squares) in milk fat during the first 21 weeks of lactation in dairy cows.

The proportion of polyunsaturated fatty acids (PUFA) was relatively constant from week 1 up to week 21 p.p. (2.6 to 2.8 g/100 g FAME; Figure 34). These results are confirmed by Stoop et al. (2009). Due to the increased adipose tissue mobilization during the NEB in early lactation, preformed FA concentrations (sum of fatty acids > C16) were greatest in week 1 p.p. (46.1 ± 1.4 g/100g FAME) and decreased in a similar pattern as reported by Kay et al. (2005) to 32.0 ± 1.0 g/100g FAME in week 12 p.p. (Table 7). Oleic acid (C18:1,9c) is the predominant FA in adipocytes and primarily released through lipolysis during a NEB (Rukkwamsuk et al., 2000). These long-chain fatty acids (preformed fatty acids) are incorporated into milk fat (Palmquist et al., 1993) and inhibit the de novo synthesis of short-chain fatty acids by the mammary gland (Bauman and Davis, 1974).The observed increase in short-chain fatty acids with progressing lactation in the present study is consistent with the decreasing adipose tissue mobilization at around week 4 to 6 p.p. (Garnsworthy and Huggett, 1992; Palmquist et al., 1993). Palmquist et al. (1993) reported that synthesis of C4:0 is not inhibited at all because of its origin from two pathways independent of the inhibitable acetyl-coenzyme A carboxylase pathway. These are preformed 4-carbon units (beta-hydroxybutyrate) and the formation by condensation of two acetyl units. Contrary to the findings of Stoop et al. (2009), trans fatty acids slightly increased with improved energy status of dairy cows from 1.4 ± 0.1 g/100g FAME (week 1 p.p.) up to 1.7 ± 0.0 g/100g FAME in week 21 p.p. of the present study (Table 7). The proportion of CLA in milk fat remained constant from week 1 to 12 p.p. (0.37 to 0.39 g/100g FAME) and increased slightly thereafter up to week 21 p.p. (0.5 ± 0.0 g/100g FAME), whereas the ratio of n6:n3 fatty acids decreased from week 12 (5.1 ± 0.2) to 21 p.p. (4.3 ± 0.1; Table 7). Milk fatty acids out of the de novo synthesis (< C16) in the present study increased from week 1 p.p. (22.6 ± 1.1 g/100g FAME) up to week 12 p.p. (30.4 ± 0.6 g/100g FAME) along with total C16 fatty acids (Table 7) in agreement with Palmquist et al. (1993) and Kay et al. (2005). Although the de novo synthesized fatty acids comprise approximately 40% by weight over the entire lactation, preformed fatty acids contribute a larger portion of the total FA in early lactation (Kay et al., 2005). Garnsworthy et al. (2006) concluded that stage of lactation does not affect the relative incorporation of de novo synthesized and preformed fatty acids when the composition of diets remains constant. Because of the same feeding regimen in the present study, changes in milk FA profile regarding de novo synthesized and preformed fatty acids therefore reflect changes in energy status of dairy cows.

Changes in milk FA composition during feed-restriction and subsequent realimentation

Data on the effects of a specific induced NEB on milk fat composition are scarce (Stoop et al. 2009). The present study contributes to increase knowledge in this respect. Milk FA profile of control-fed cows in the present study was stable during feed-restriction (period 2) and the subsequent realimentation (period 3) (Table 8). For restricted cows, the proportion of most fatty acids ≤ C16:0 (e.g., C6:0, C10:0, C10:1, C12:0, C14:0, C16:0) was decreased during the NEB induced by feed-restriction compared to week 0 of period 2, whereas preformed fatty acids, especially C17:1,9c, C18:0 and C18:1,9c arising from body fat mobilization increased markedly during feed-restriction (Table 8). These changes occurred rapidly within the first week of feed-restriction (on average 3 days distance between the start of feed-restriction and the next milking sample) and disappeared completely within one week of realimentation (4 days on average). The proportion of CLA in milk fat of feed-restricted cows was elevated in week 1 of period 2 (0.5 ± 0.0 g/100 g FAME) compared to week 0 of period 2 (0.4 ± 0.0 g/100g FAME) and adjusted immediately to initial values (Table 8). The n6:n3-ratio steadily decreased for restricted cows during period 2 from 4.4 ± 0.3 (week 0) until 3.7 ± 0.2 (week 3) and increased again during subsequent realimentation (Table 8). Despite the maintenance of the deliberately induced NEB by feed-restriction at a relatively constant level, fatty acids showed a tendency during the NEB to adjust towards the initial levels before feed-restriction. The pattern of decreasing short-chain fatty acids and increase of long-chain fatty acids during an induced NEB was reported in an earlier study of Luick and Smith (1963). The proportions of C15:0iso, C15:0anteiso, C16:1,9c, C17:0iso or C17:0 were not affected by feed-restriction in the present study (Table 8). During feed-restriction (period 2), SFA decreased from initially 75.3 ± 0.4 g/100g FAME (week 0) to 69.5 ± 1.0 g/100g FAME (week 1), while MUFA (especially C18:1,9c) increased for restricted cows from 20.2 ± 0.3 g/100g FAME (week 0) to 25.6 ± 0.9 g/100g FAME (week 1; Figure 35). PUFA were relatively stable during period 2 and the following realimentation period in feed-restricted cows (2.3 to 2.8 g/100g FAME; Figure 35).

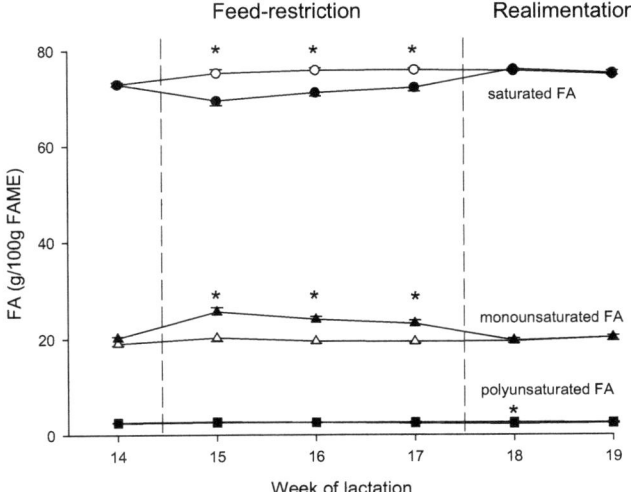

Figure 35. Changes in saturated FA (circles), monounsaturated FA (triangles) and polyunsaturated FA (squares) in milk fat of feed-restricted cows (filled symbols) and control cows (empty symbols) during feed-restriction (week 15 to 17 post partum) and subsequent realimentation (week 18 to 19 post partum). Stars indicate a significant difference between the groups ($P < 0.05$).

Table 8. Changes in milk fatty acid (FA) composition for feed-restricted and control cows during feed-restriction and realimentation. Differences over time within group are marked with different superscripts, differences between the groups within week are marked with * ($P < 0.05$).

Week	Restricted Group (n=20)					
	Feed-restriction				Realimentation	
	0	1	2	3	1	2
FA (g/100g FAME)						
4:0	2.97 ± 0.07	3.03 ± 0.10	3.15 ± 0.11	3.17 ± 0.12	3.21 ± 0.13	3.13 ± 0.11
6:0	2.35^a ± 0.06	$2.15*^b$ ± 0.04	2.30^{ab} ± 0.06	2.32^{ab} ± 0.07	2.45^a ± 0.08	2.42^a ± 0.03
8:0	1.51^a ± 0.04	$1.29*^b$ ± 0.03	$1.36*^b$ ± 0.03	$1.38*^b$ ± 0.04	1.53^a ± 0.04	1.54^a ± 0.04
10:0	3.60^a ± 0.08	$2.79*^b$ ± 0.10	$2.96*^b$ ± 0.09	$3.05*^b$ ± 0.10	3.59^a ± 0.10	3.64^a ± 0.10
10:1	0.36^a ± 0.01	$0.27*^c$ ± 0.01	$0.29*^{bc}$ ± 0.01	0.32^b ± 0.01	$0.39*^a$ ± 0.01	$0.38*^a$ ± 0.01
11:0	0.13^a ± 0.01	$0.05*^c$ ± 0.01	$0.05*^c$ ± 0.01	$0.06*^c$ ± 0.01	0.10^b ± 0.01	0.12^{ab} ± 0.01
12:0	4.27^a ± 0.08	$3.18*^b$ ± 0.13	$3.32*^b$ ± 0.13	$3.49*^b$ ± 0.13	4.34^a ± 0.13	4.37^a ± 0.13
12:1	0.11^b ± 0.00	$0.07*^d$ ± 0.00	$0.08*^{cd}$ ± 0.00	0.09^c ± 0.01	$0.13*^a$ ± 0.01	$0.12*^a$ ± 0.00
13:0	0.19^a ± 0.02	$0.11*^c$ ± 0.01	$0.11*^c$ ± 0.01	$0.11*^c$ ± 0.01	0.16^b ± 0.01	0.18^{ab} ± 0.01
14:0iso	0.08^b ± 0.01	0.09^{ab} ± 0.01	0.10^a ± 0.01	0.10^{ab} ± 0.00	$0.08*^b$ ± 0.01	0.09^b ± 0.01
14:0	12.38^a ± 0.16	$10.95*^b$ ± 0.29	$11.38*^b$ ± 0.22	11.46^b ± 0.22	12.26^a ± 0.21	12.29^a ± 0.18
14:1,9c	1.40^{ab} ± 0.13	1.14^b ± 0.10	1.21^{ab} ± 0.10	1.27^{ab} ± 0.08	1.50^a ± 0.12	1.50^a ± 0.14
15:0iso	0.21^{ab} ± 0.01	0.23^a ± 0.01	0.23^a ± 0.01	0.23^{ab} ± 0.01	$0.20*^b$ ± 0.01	0.21^b ± 0.01
15:0anteiso	0.45 ± 0.01	0.41 ± 0.02	0.43 ± 0.01	0.43 ± 0.01	0.43 ± 0.01	0.44 ± 0.01
15:0	1.44^a ± 0.09	$1.00*^b$ ± 0.05	$1.01*^b$ ± 0.05	1.04^b ± 0.04	1.26^a ± 0.06	1.37^a ± 0.09
16:0iso	0.18^b ± 0.01	0.24^a ± 0.01	0.24^a ± 0.01	0.22^{ab} ± 0.01	0.20^b ± 0.01	$0.19*^b$ ± 0.01
16:0	36.14^{ab} ± 0.61	$32.63*^d$ ± 0.67	$33.51*^{cd}$ ± 0.69	$34.58*^{bc}$ ± 0.74	37.84^a ± 0.62	36.03^{ab} ± 0.51
16:1,9c	1.86 ± 0.08	1.94 ± 0.09	1.91 ± 0.08	1.93 ± 0.08	2.06 ± 0.09	1.95 ± 0.08
17:0iso	0.24 ± 0.03	0.25 ± 0.02	0.23 ± 0.02	0.23 ± 0.02	0.21 ± 0.03	0.23 ± 0.03
17:0anteiso	0.35^{cd} ± 0.01	$0.40*^a$ ± 0.01	0.38^{ab} ± 0.01	0.37^{bc} ± 0.01	0.33^d ± 0.01	0.34^{cd} ± 0.01
17:0	0.39 ± 0.02	0.39 ± 0.01	0.37 ± 0.02	0.36 ± 0.02	0.34 ± 0.02	0.36 ± 0.02
17:1,9c	0.21^b ± 0.01	$0.28*^a$ ± 0.02	$0.26*^a$ ± 0.01	$0.25*^a$ ± 0.02	0.21^b ± 0.01	0.21^b ± 0.01
18:0	8.22^b ± 0.19	$10.09*^a$ ± 0.22	$9.86*^a$ ± 0.29	$9.46*^a$ ± 0.35	$7.44*^b$ ± 0.32	8.19^b ± 0.25
18:1,9t	0.41^{ab} ± 0.01	$0.43*^a$ ± 0.01	0.44^a ± 0.01	0.43^{ab} ± 0.01	0.39^b ± 0.01	0.42^{ab} ± 0.01
18:1,11t	1.10^{ab} ± 0.05	1.18^{ab} ± 0.05	1.21^a ± 0.06	1.20^a ± 0.05	1.05^b ± 0.05	1.10^{ab} ± 0.05
18:1,9c	15.27^c ± 0.25	$20.89*^a$ ± 0.85	$19.29*^{ab}$ ± 0.61	$18.42*^b$ ± 0.67	14.58^c ± 0.43	15.27^c ± 0.36

Table 8. (continued)

Control Group (n=20)					
Feed-restriction				Realimentation	
0	1	2	3	1	2
3.08	3.10	3.17	3.10	3.10	3.03
± 0.08	± 0.05	± 0.12	± 0.07	± 0.07	± 0.05
2.41	2.38	2.46	2.40	2.41	2.34
± 0.04	± 0.04	± 0.06	± 0.05	± 0.05	± 0.03
1.53	1.49	1.55	1.51	1.52	1.47
± 0.03	± 0.04	± 0.03	± 0.04	± 0.03	± 0.03
3.73	3.54	3.70	3.61	3.62	3.48
± 0.09	± 0.11	± 0.09	± 0.11	± 0.10	± 0.08
0.34	0.32	0.33	0.32	0.33	0.32
± 0.01	± 0.01	± 0.01	± 0.01	± 0.02	± 0.01
0.12	0.10	0.11	0.10	0.11	0.10
± 0.01	± 0.01	± 0.01	± 0.01	± 0.01	± 0.01
4.47	4.16	4.35	4.27	4.28	4.10
± 0.13	± 0.15	± 0.12	± 0.14	± 0.13	± 0.10
0.10	0.09	0.10	0.10	0.10	0.10
± 0.00	± 0.01	± 0.00	± 0.00	± 0.01	± 0.00
0.18	0.16	0.17	0.16	0.17	0.16
± 0.01	± 0.01	± 0.01	± 0.01	± 0.01	± 0.01
0.09	0.09	0.09	0.10	0.11	0.10
± 0.01	± 0.01	± 0.01	± 0.01	± 0.01	± 0.01
12.36	12.00	12.20	12.18	12.29	12.03
± 0.19	± 0.28	± 0.22	± 0.24	± 0.22	± 0.25
1.13	1.07	1.08	1.07	1.14	1.51
± 0.05	± 0.06	± 0.05	± 0.05	± 0.06	± 0.12
0.21	0.22	0.21	0.22	0.23	0.22
± 0.01	± 0.01	± 0.01	± 0.01	± 0.01	± 0.01
0.43	0.43	0.43	0.44	0.45	0.44
± 0.01	± 0.01	± 0.01	± 0.01	± 0.01	± 0.01
1.29	1.21	1.26	1.22	1.24	1.22
± 0.07	± 0.07	± 0.09	± 0.07	± 0.07	± 0.07
0.21	0.21	0.22	0.22	0.22	0.23
± 0.01	± 0.01	± 0.01	± 0.02	± 0.01	± 0.02
37.35	36.52	36.38	36.75	36.43	36.52
± 0.64	± 0.75	± 0.73	± 0.55	± 0.69	± 0.78
1.85	1.86	1.80	1.78	1.84	1.83
± 0.08	± 0.11	± 0.08	± 0.08	± 0.08	± 0.10
0.19	0.19	0.18	0.19	0.18	0.19
± 0.03	± 0.02	± 0.02	± 0.02	± 0.02	± 0.02
0.35	0.36	0.35	0.36	0.36	0.36
± 0.01	± 0.01	± 0.01	± 0.01	± 0.01	± 0.01
0.37	0.37	0.36	0.36	0.36	0.36
± 0.01	± 0.01	± 0.01	± 0.01	± 0.01	± 0.01
0.20	0.21	0.19	0.19	0.20	0.19
± 0.01	± 0.01	± 0.01	± 0.01	± 0.01	± 0.01
8.02	8.56	8.51	8.56	8.53	8.49
± 0.25	± 0.41	± 0.33	± 0.24	± 0.36	± 0.39
0.39	0.39	0.40	0.40	0.41	0.41
± 0.01	± 0.01	± 0.01	± 0.01	± 0.01	± 0.01
1.07^b	1.06^b	1.13^{ab}	1.15^{ab}	1.18^{ab}	1.20^a
± 0.05	± 0.05	± 0.05	± 0.04	± 0.05	± 0.06
14.42	15.69	15.01	14.99	15.04	15.07
± 0.34	± 0.70	± 0.45	± 0.34	± 0.36	± 0.51

Table 8. (continued)

Week	Restricted Group (n=20)					
	Feed-restriction				Realimentation	
	0	1	2	3	1	2
FA (g/100g FAME)						
18:1,c11	0.65[ab] ± 0.04	0.73[a] ± 0.04	0.69[ab] ± 0.03	0.62[bc] ± 0.03	0.51[d] ± 0.03	0.56[cd] ± 0.03
18:1,c12	0.29 ± 0.01	0.27 ± 0.01	0.28 ± 0.01	0.27 ± 0.01	0.28 ± 0.01	0.29 ± 0.01
18:2,9c,12c	1.81[ab] ± 0.06	1.90[a] ± 0.07	1.75[ab] ± 0.04	1.64[bc] ± 0.05	1.59*[c] ± 0.05	1.67[bc] ± 0.06
18:3,9c,12c,15c	0.39[abc] ± 0.02	0.42[ab] ± 0.02	0.44[a] ± 0.02	0.41[abc] ± 0.02	0.37[bc] ± 0.02	0.37[c] ± 0.02
18:2,9c,11t	0.41 ± 0.02	0.46* ± 0.02	0.46 ± 0.02	0.45 ± 0.02	0.42 ± 0.02	0.42 ± 0.02
18:2,10t,12c	0.02 ± 0.01	0.03 ± 0.01	0.03 ± 0.01	0.03 ± 0.01	0.02 ± 0.01	0.02 ± 0.01
20:0	0.10[bc] ± 0.01	0.11[a] ± 0.01	0.11[a] ± 0.01	0.11[ab] ± 0.01	0.09[c] ± 0.01	0.09[bc] ± 0.01
20:1,11c	0.04[bc] ± 0.00	0.05*[a] ± 0.00	0.05*[a] ± 0.00	0.04[ab] ± 0.00	0.03[c] ± 0.00	0.03[c] ± 0.00
20:2,11c,14c	0.03[bc] ± 0.00	0.04[a] ± 0.00	0.03[ab] ± 0.00	0.03[ab] ± 0.00	0.03*[c] ± 0.00	0.03[bc] ± 0.00
21:0	0.03 ± 0.01	0.03 ± 0.01	0.03 ± 0.00	0.03 ± 0.00	0.02 ± 0.00	0.02 ± 0.00
20:3,8c,11c,14c	0.15[a] ± 0.01	0.15[a] ± 0.01	0.13[ab] ± 0.01	0.13[ab] ± 0.01	0.11*[b] ± 0.01	0.12[b] ± 0.01
20:4,5c,8c,11c,14c	0.13[ab] ± 0.01	0.14[a] ± 0.01	0.13[ab] ± 0.01	0.12[ab] ± 0.01	0.10[b] ± 0.01	0.11[ab] ± 0.01
20:5,5c,8c,11c,14c,17c	0.04[ab] ± 0.00	0.04[ab] ± 0.00	0.05[a] ± 0.00	0.04[ab] ± 0.00	0.04[b] ± 0.00	0.04[ab] ± 0.00
22:0	0.06[abc] ± 0.00	0.06*[ab] ± 0.00	0.06*[a] ± 0.00	0.06[ab] ± 0.00	0.05[c] ± 0.00	0.05[bc] ± 0.00
22:5,7c,10c,13c,16c,19c	0.07 ± 0.01	0.09 ± 0.01	0.08 ± 0.01	0.08 ± 0.01	0.08 ± 0.01	0.08 ± 0.01
Summarized FA						
n6 FA	2.11[ab] ± 0.07	2.22[a] ± 0.08	2.05[bc] ± 0.05	1.92[cd] ± 0.05	1.84*[d] ± 0.05	1.94[cd] ± 0.06
n3 FA	0.50[ab] ± 0.03	0.55[ab] ± 0.03	0.56[a] ± 0.03	0.53[ab] ± 0.02	0.49[b] ± 0.02	0.49[b] ± 0.02
n6:n3-ratio	4.42[a] ± 0.28	4.16[ab] ± 0.18	3.76*[b] ± 0.16	3.69*[b] ± 0.17	3.88[ab] ± 0.19	4.07[ab] ± 0.16
CLA	0.43[b] ± 0.02	0.50*[a] ± 0.02	0.49[ab] ± 0.03	0.47[ab] ± 0.02	0.44[ab] ± 0.02	0.44[ab] ± 0.02
trans FA	1.51[ab] ± 0.06	1.61[ab] ± 0.06	1.65[a] ± 0.07	1.63[a] ± 0.06	1.44[b] ± 0.06	1.52[ab] ± 0.06
de novo syn. FA	31.44[a] ± 0.41	26.78*[c] ± 0.63	27.99[bc] ± 0.55	28.51*[b] ± 0.58	31.61[a] ± 0.57	31.80[a] ± 0.52
total C16 FA	38.18[ab] ± 0.66	34.80*[d] ± 0.67	35.66*[cd] ± 0.71	36.73*[bc] ± 0.77	40.10[a] ± 0.68	38.17[b] ± 0.56
preformed FA	30.38[c] ± 0.42	38.42*[a] ± 0.97	36.36*[ab] ± 0.87	34.76*[b] ± 0.99	28.30[c] ± 0.78	30.03[c] ± 0.65

Table 8. (continued)

	Control Group (n=20)					
	Feed-restriction				Realimentation	
	0	1	2	3	1	2
	0.68 ± 0.11	0.71 ± 0.09	0.70 ± 0.10	0.68 ± 0.11	0.56 ± 0.04	0.65 ± 0.09
	0.27^{ab} ± 0.01	0.27^{b} ± 0.01	0.29^{ab} ± 0.01	0.29^{ab} ± 0.01	0.31^{a} ± 0.01	0.29^{ab} ± 0.01
	1.77 ± 0.05	1.83 ± 0.05	1.82 ± 0.06	1.79 ± 0.05	1.79 ± 0.06	1.77 ± 0.06
	0.37 ± 0.02	0.38 ± 0.01	0.39 ± 0.02	0.40 ± 0.02	0.41 ± 0.03	0.38 ± 0.02
	0.39^{b} ± 0.02	0.40^{ab} ± 0.02	0.41^{ab} ± 0.02	0.43^{ab} ± 0.02	0.44^{a} ± 0.02	0.45^{a} ± 0.02
	0.03 ± 0.01	0.03 ± 0.01	0.03 ± 0.01	0.03 ± 0.01	0.03 ± 0.01	0.03 ± 0.01
	0.09 ± 0.01	0.09 ± 0.01	0.10 ± 0.01	0.10 ± 0.01	0.10 ± 0.01	0.10 ± 0.01
	0.04 ± 0.00	0.04 ± 0.00	0.04 ± 0.00	0.04 ± 0.00	0.04 ± 0.00	0.03 ± 0.00
	0.03 ± 0.00	0.03 ± 0.00	0.03 ± 0.00	0.03 ± 0.00	0.03 ± 0.00	0.03 ± 0.00
	0.03 ± 0.01	0.04 ± 0.01	0.04 ± 0.01	0.03 ± 0.01	0.04 ± 0.01	0.04 ± 0.01
	0.13 ± 0.01	0.13 ± 0.01	0.13 ± 0.01	0.14 ± 0.01	0.14 ± 0.01	0.14 ± 0.01
	0.12 ± 0.01	0.12 ± 0.01	0.12 ± 0.01	0.12 ± 0.01	0.12 ± 0.01	0.12 ± 0.01
	0.04 ± 0.00	0.04 ± 0.00	0.04 ± 0.00	0.04 ± 0.00	0.04 ± 0.00	0.04 ± 0.00
	0.05 ± 0.00	0.05 ± 0.00	0.05 ± 0.00	0.05 ± 0.00	0.05 ± 0.00	0.05 ± 0.00
	0.06 ± 0.01	0.07 ± 0.01	0.07 ± 0.01	0.06 ± 0.01	0.07 ± 0.01	0.06 ± 0.01
Summarized FA						
	2.05 ± 0.06	2.11 ± 0.06	2.11 ± 0.07	2.09 ± 0.06	2.09 ± 0.07	2.06 ± 0.06
	0.48 ± 0.02	0.49 ± 0.02	0.50 ± 0.02	0.51 ± 0.03	0.52 ± 0.03	0.49 ± 0.03
	4.46 ± 0.20	4.44 ± 0.19	4.32 ± 0.18	4.28 ± 0.19	4.28 ± 0.24	4.35 ± 0.18
	0.42^{b} ± 0.02	0.43^{ab} ± 0.02	0.44^{ab} ± 0.02	0.46^{ab} ± 0.02	0.47^{ab} ± 0.02	0.48^{a} ± 0.02
	1.45^{b} ± 0.05	1.45^{b} ± 0.05	1.52^{ab} ± 0.06	1.55^{ab} ± 0.05	1.59^{ab} ± 0.06	1.62^{a} ± 0.07
	31.48 ± 0.34	30.37 ± 0.63	31.21 ± 0.42	30.80 ± 0.49	31.09 ± 0.48	30.93 ± 0.71
	39.41 ± 0.67	38.58 ± 0.80	38.39 ± 0.77	38.76 ± 0.58	38.49 ± 0.73	38.58 ± 0.83
	29.11 ± 0.57	31.05 ± 1.10	30.40 ± 0.79	30.44 ± 0.50	30.41 ± 0.71	30.49 ± 1.02

Leiber et al. (2005) reported that mobilization of body fat is typical for alpine pastured cows and that the elevated C18:3,9c,12c,15c concentration in milk fat could originate from body fat and grass intake on pasture. Leiber et al. (2005) suggested that in response to the nutritional energy deficiency during the alpine period, the rumen microbial capacity for biohydrogenation might be reduced and more C18:3 remained available for absorption. The proportion of C18:3 did not differ between the two groups during feed-restriction in the present study (Table 9). Luick and Smith (1963) examined whether changes in milk FA composition during energy-restriction are caused by a decreased synthesis of short-chain fatty acids or by an increased incorporation of long-chain fatty acids absorbed from the plasma. According to Luick and Smith (1963), the failure to utilize beta-hydroxybutyrate occurs when its concentration in plasma is elevated, i.e., during fasting and ketosis. This in turn, accounts for the relatively high levels of oleic-acid found in milk fat of fasting and ketotic cows (Luick and Smith, 1963) as observed in the present study. Although less in their extent, milk fatty acids clearly showed a similar pattern during a deliberately induced NEB by feed-restriction at around 100 DIM compared to the NEB in early lactation. Compared to milk of dairy cows in a positive energy balance (week 14 p.p.), for several fatty acids proportions changed up to 80% (e.g., C17:1,9c; C18:1,9c) during the NEB in early lactation and during the deliberately induced NEB by feed-restriction. This increase was independent from the proportion in milk fat (C17:1,9c is represented at 0.2 g/100g FAME and C18:1,9c at 15.3 g/100g FAME in week 14 p.p.).

Mobilization of adipose tissue precedes ketosis development (Reist et al., 2003). With regard to this fact, van Haelst et al. (2008) determined whether concentrations of specific fatty acids in milk fat are suitable for the early detection of subclinical ketosis. Van Haelst et al. (2008) suggested the elevated proportion of C18:1,9c as an interesting trait for prediction of subclinical ketosis, particularly since this FA was elevated in milk fat before diagnosis of ketosis. As milk fatty acids changed with altering energy status, it is obvious to identify milk fatty acids indicating a NEB in dairy cows independent of their lactational stage. Therefore, correlations between milk fatty acids and the energy balance were calculated. In the present study, the correlation between energy status and the proportion of C18:1,9c in milk fat of 5 cows with the most negative EB in week 1 p.p. (-80.2 MJ NEL/d) was 0.62. Also the correlation between EB and C18:1,9c for feed-restricted cows with the highest NEB in the first week of feed-restriction (-83.2 MJ NEL/d) was 0.92. Therefore, an elevated proportion of C18:1,9c in milk fat can be confirmed to be a suitable marker for a NEB. The correlation between energy status and other single fatty acids during the NEB in early lactation and during the deliberately induced NEB ranged from 0.71 to 0.96. However, the low proportion and relatively high variation in changed fatty acids (e.g., C11:0; C12:1; Table 9) restrict the predictive value of these fatty acids to indicate a NEB although changes were significant between energy-restricted and control cows. The correlation between energy status and groups of fatty acids was higher in cows with a more intense NEB during feed-restriction that ranged from 0.92 up to 0.98 for SFA, MUFA, de novo synthesized and preformed fatty acids. The higher proportion of these summarized fatty acids in milk fat makes their changes a more appropriate tool reflecting energy status in dairy cows compared to single fatty acids represented at a low concentration. However, these findings only apply to constant feeding conditions.

58 Results and Discussion

4. Conclusions

Following conclusions out of the present study regarding adaptation of dairy cows to a NEB at two different stages of lactation can be drawn:

- Dairy cows experienced a clear lactation-induced NEB during the first weeks after parturition as a result of lower energy intake by feed than energy requirements for maintenance and lactation.
- The deliberately induced NEB by feed-restriction at around 100 DIM was higher compared to the lactation-induced NEB post partum.
- The balance of ACP followed the pattern of EB during the experimental periods and was negative in early lactation and during the feed-restriction period.
- Milk production showed highest priority after parturition, where milk yield increased despite the lactation-induced NEB.
- During the nutrition-induced NEB, milk yield immediately decreased though changes were small and completely recovered in the subsequent realimentation period.
- During the deliberately induced NEB, only milk protein was decreased, though changes were small. The milk fat-protein ratio was elevated during both periods of a NEB in the present study and therefore suitable to indicate a NEB.
- Both periods of a NEB in the present study were accompanied by mobilization of body reserves. Body weight, BCS, backfat thickness and the muscle diameter of the longissimus dorsi muscle decreased during the NEB in early and mid lactation. Except for BFT, all condition parameters fully recovered during the realimentation period.
- Plasma glucose concentration was markedly reduced after parturition and only slightly decreased during the feed-restriction period. Plasma NEFA and BHBA concentrations were elevated during both stages of the NEB, though changes were marginal during the deliberately induced NEB compared to the lactation-induced NEB. In the realimentation period, plasma metabolites were not altered anymore.
- Endocrine factors and liver gene expressions of constituents of the somatotropic axis and insulin system were markedly affected by the NEB in early lactation. However, changes during the deliberately induced NEB by feed-restriction were less pronounced. The adaptation of these parameters to a NEB was either same directed, opposite directed or unchanged when comparing the two lactational stages of the NEB (Table 10). Table 10 shows the different reactions in bold type.

Table 9. Direction of adaptation of endocrine factors and liver gene expression parameters during the two stages of a NEB. Different adaptations are given in bold type.

	NEB induced by lactation	NEB induced by feed-restriction
Endocrine factors in plasma		
GH	⬆	=
IGF-I	↓	↓
Insulin	⬇	=
Leptin	↓	↓
T$_3$	⬇	=
T$_4$	⬇	=
Gene expressions in liver		
GHR 1A	⬇	=
IGF-I	⬇	=
IGF-IR	=	⬆
IGFBP-1	↑	↑
IGFBP-2	↑	↑
IGFBP-3	⬇	⬆
INSR	↑	↑

- Endocrine factors fully recovered during the realimentation period.
- Possibly the expression of IGFBP-3 is the key regulatory element in the different adaptation of the somatotropic axis to a NEB. Plasma IGFBPs have to be measured to confirm this hypothesis.
- Milk fatty acids responded in a same directed way to the NEB in early lactation and the NEB induced by feed-restriction.
- Under constant feeding conditions, milk fatty acids closely correlate with energy status of dairy cows.
- Oleic acid as a single FA and the summarized fatty acids (SFA, MUFA, de novo synthesized and preformed fatty acids) are suitable to identify a NEB under a constant feeding regimen.

5. References

Bauman, D. E. 2000. Regulation of nutrient partitioning during lactation: Homeostasis and homeorhesis revisited. In: Ruminant Physiology. Digestion, metabolism, growth and reproduction. Ed. P. B. Cronje, Commonwealth Agricultural Bureau International, 2000, 311-328.

Bauman, D. E., and W. B. Currie. 1980. Partitioning of nutrients during pregnancy and lactation: a review of mechanisms involving homeostasis homeorhesis. J. Dairy Sci. 63:1514-1529.

Bauman, D. E., and C. L. Davis. 1974. Biosynthesis of milk fat. Page 31 in: Lactation – A comprehensive treatise. Vol. 2. Larson BL & Smith VR, ed. Academic Press, New York, NY.

Bauman, D. E., and J. M. Elliot. 1983. Control of nutrient partitioning in lactating ruminants. Pages 437-468 in: Biochemistry of Lactation. T. B. Mepham, ed. Elsevier Science Publishers, Amsterdam, the Netherlands.

Bauman, D. E., J. H. Eisemann, and W. B. Currie. 1982. Hormonal effects on partitioning of nutrients for tissue growth: role of growth hormone and prolactin. Fed. Proc. 41:2538-2544.

Baxter, C. F., M. Kleiber, and A. L. Black. 1956. The blood precursors of lactose as studied with 14C-labeled metabolites in intact dairy cows. Biochim. Biophys. Acta 21:277-285.

Baxter, R. C. 1993. IGF binding protein-3 and the acid-labile subunit: formation of the ternary complex in vitro and in vivo. Adv. Exp. Med. Biol. 343:237-244.

Bell, A. W. 1995. Regulation of organic nutrient metabolism during transition from late pregnancy to early lactation. J. Anim. Sci. 73:2804-2819.

Bell, A. W., and D. E. Bauman. 1997. Adaptations of glucose metabolism during pregnancy and lactation. J. Mammary Gland Biol. Neopl. 2:265-278.

Berg, J. M., J. L. Tymoczko, and S. Lubert. 2006. Biochemistry. 6th ed. W. H. Freeman, New York, USA.

Bertoni, G., E. Trevisi, and R. Lombardelli. 2009. Some new aspects of nutrition, health conditions and fertility of intensively reared dairy cows. Ital. J. Anim. Sci. 8:491-518.

Björntorp, P., S. Edström, J. G. Kral, K. Lundholm, E. Presta, D. Walks, and M.-U. Yang. 1982. Refeeding after fasting in the rat: energy substrate fluxes and replenishment of energy stores. Am. J. Clin. Nutr. 36:450-456.

Bligh, E. G., and W. J. Dyer. 1959. A rapid method of total lipid extraction and purification. Can. J. Biochem. Physiol. 37:911-917.

Block, S. S., W. R. Butler, R. A. Ehrhardt, A. W. Bell, M. E. van Amburgh, and Y. R. Boisclair. 2001. Decreased concentration of plasma leptin in peiparturient dairy cows is caused by negative energy balance. J. Endocrinol. 171:339-348.

Block, S. S., R. P. Rhoads, D. E. Bauman, R. A. Ehrhardt, M. A. McGuire, B. A. Crooker, J. M. Griinari, T. R. Mackle, W. J. Weber, M. E. van Amburgh, and Y. R. Boisclair. 2003a. Demonstration of a role for insulin in the regulation of leptin in lactating dairy cows. J. Dairy Sci. 86:3508-3515.

Block, S. S., J. M. Smith, R. A. Ehrhardt, M. C. Diaz, R. P. Rhoads, M. E. van Amburgh, and Y. R. Boisclair. 2003b. Nutritional and developmental regulation of plasma leptin in dairy cattle. J. Dairy Sci. 86:3206-3214.

Blum, J. W., P. Kunz, H. Leuenberger, K. Gautschi, and M. Keller. 1983. Thyroid hormones, blood plasma metabolites and haematological parameters in relationship to milk yield in dairy cows. Anim. Prod. 36:93-104.

Boisclair, Y. R., S. R. Wesolowski, J. W. Kim, and R. A. Ehrhardt. 2006. Roles of growth hormone and leptin in the periparturient dairy cow. In: Ruminant Physiology. Digestion, metabolism and impact of nutrition on gene expression, immunology and stress. Ed. Sejrsen, K., T. Hvelupund, and M. O. Nielsen. Wageningen Academic Publishers, the Netherlands, 2006, 327-344.

Bradford, B. J., and M. S. Allen. 2008. Negative energy balance increases peripheral ghrelin and growth hormone concentrations in lactating dairy cows. Domest. Anim. Endocrinol. 34:196-203.

Breier, B. H. 1999. Regulation of protein- and energy metabolism by the somatotropic axis. Domest. Anim. Endocrinol. 17:209-218.

Bruckmaier, R. M., L. Gregoretti, F. Jans, D. Faissler, and J. W. Blum. 1998a. Longissimus dorsi muscle diameter, backfat thickness, body condition scores and skinfold values related to metabolic and endocrine traits in lactating dairy cows fed crystalline fat or free fatty acids. J. Vet. Med. Ser. A 45:397-410.

Bruckmaier, R. M., E. Lehmann, D. Hugi, H. M. Hammon, and J. W. Blum. 1998b. Ultrasonic measurement of longissimus dorsi muscle and backfat, associated with metabolic and endocrine traits, during fattening of intact and castrated male cattle. Livest. Prod. Sci. 53:123-134.

Bruckmaier, R. M., and H. A. van Dorland. 2010. Advantage of complementary liver transcripts to understand metabolic biodiversity in dairy cows? In: Energy and protein metabolism and nutrition, EAAP publication No. 127, 2010, 3rd EAAP ISEP, Parma, Italy, 6-10 September 2010 (ed. G. Matteo Corvetto), 469-478.

Butler, S. T., A. L. Marr, S. H. Pelton, R. P. Radcliff, M. C. Lucy, and W. R. Butler. 2003. Insulin restores GH responsiveness during lactation-induced negative energy balance in dairy cattle: effects on expression of IGF-I and GH receptor 1A. J. Endocrinol. 176:205-217.

Butler, W. R., and R. D. Smith. 1989. Interrelationships between energy balance and postpartum reproductive function in dairy cattle. J. Dairy Sci. 72:767-783.

Cannon, W. B. 1929. Organization for physiological homeostasis. Physiol. Rev. 9:399-431.

Carlson, D. B., N. B. Litherland, H. M. Dann, J. C. Woodworth, and J. K. Drackley. 2006. Metabolic effects of abomasal L-carnitine infusion and feed restriction in lactating Holstein cows. J. Dairy Sci. 89:4819-4834.

Carriquiry, M., W. J. Weber, S. C. Fahrenkrug, and B. A. Crooker. 2009. Hepatic gene expression in multiparous Holstein cows treated with bovine somatotropin and fed n-3 fatty acids in early lactation. J. Dairy Sci. 92:4889-4900.

Chagas, L. M., M. C. Lucy, P. J. Back, D. Blache, J. M. Lee, P. J. S. Gore, A. J. Sheanan, and J. R. Roche. 2009. Insulin resistance in divergent strains of Holstein-Friesian dairy cows offered fresh pasture and increasing amounts of concentrate in early lactation. J. Dairy Sci. 92:216-222.

Chilliard, Y., M. Bonnet, C. Delavaud, Y. Faulconnier, C. Leroux, J. Djiane, and F. Bocquier. 2001. Leptin in ruminants. Gene expression in adipose tissue and mammary gland, and regulation of plasma concentration. Domest. Anim. Endocrinol. 21:271-295.

Cnaan, A., N. M. Laird, and P. Slasor. 1997. Tutorial in biostatistics: using the general linear mixed model to analyse unbalanced repeated measures and longitudinal data. Statistics in Medicine. 16:2349-2380.

Collard, B. L., P. J. Boettcher, J. C. M. Dekkers, D. petitclerc, and L. R. Schaeffer. 2000. Relationships between energy balance and health traits of dairy cattle in early lactation. J. Dairy Sci. 83:2683-2690.

Delavaud, C., A. Ferlay, Y. Faulconnier, F. Bocquier, G. Kann, and Y. Chilliard. 2002. Plasma leptin concentration in adult cattle: effects of breed, adiposity, feeding level, and meal intake. J. Anim. Sci. 80:1317-1328.

DLG. 1997. DLG-Futterwerttabellen Wiederkäuer. 7. überarb. und erw. Aufl., DLG-Verlag. Frankfurt am Main.

Doepel, L., H. Lapierre, and J. J. Kennelly. 2002. Peripartum performance and metabolism of dairy cows in response to prepartum energy and protein intake. J. Dairy Sci. 85:2315-2334.

Edmonson, A. J., I. J. Lean, L. D. Weaver, T. Farver, and G. Webster. 1989. A body condition scoring chart for Holstein dairy cows. J. Dairy Sci. 72:68-78.

Etherton, T. D., and D. E. Bauman. 1998. Biology of somatotropin in growth and lactation of domestic animals. Physiol. Rev. 78:745-761.

FAO. 2011. Food and Agriculture Organization of the United Nations, FAOSTAT, FAO Statistics Division 2011.

Fenwick, M. A., R. Fitzpatrick, D. A. Kenny, M. G. Diskin, J. Patton, J. J. Murphy, and D. C. Wathes. 2008. Interrelationships between negative energy balance (NEB) and IGF regulation in liver of lactating dairy cows. Domest. Anim. Endocrinol. 34:31-44.

Fleiss, J. L. 1986. The design and analysis of clinical experiments. Wiley, New York.

Garnsworthy, P. C., and C. D. Huggett. 1992. The influence of the fat concentration of the diet on the response by dairy cows to body condition at calving. Anim. Prod. 54:7-13.

Garnsworthy, P. C., L. L. Masson, A. L. Lock, and T. T. Mottram. 2006. Variation of milk citrate with stage of lactation and de novo fatty acid synthesis in dairy cows. J. Dairy Sci. 89:1604-1612.

GfE (German Society of Nutrition Physiology). 2001. Empfehlungen zur Energie- und Nährstoffversorgung der Milchkühe und Aufzuchtrinder, Ausschuss für Bedarfsnormen der Gesellschaft für Ernährungsphysiologie. DLG-Verlag, Frankfurt am Main.

Goff, J. P., and R. L. Horst. 1997. Physiological changes at parturition and their relationship to metabolic disorders. J. Dairy Sci. 80:1260-1268.

Grummer, R. R. 1993. Etiology of lipid-related metabolic disorders in periparturient dairy cows. J. Dairy Sci. 76:3882-3896.

Grummer, R. R. 2007. Strategies to improve fertility of high yielding dairy farms: Management of the dry period. Theriogenology. 68, Suppl. 1:S281-288.

Grummer, R. R. 2008. Nutritional and management strategies for the prevention of fatty liver in dairy cattle. Vet. J. 176:10-20.

Hachenberg, S., C. Weinkauf, S. Hiss, and H. Sauerwein. 2007. Evaluation of classification modes potentially suitable to identify metabolic stress in healthy dairy cows during the peripartal period. J. Anim. Sci. 85:1923-1932.

Hallermayer, R. 1976. Eine Schnellmethode zur Bestimmung des Fettgehaltes in Lebensmitteln. [A rapid method to determine fat content in food]. Deutsche Lebensmittelrundschau. 10:356-359.

Hanley, J. A., and B. J. McNeil. 1982. The meaning and use of the area under the Receiver Operating Characteristics (ROC) curve. Radiology. 143:29-36.

Heuer, C., Y. H. Schukken, and P. Dobbelaar. 1999. Postpartum body condition score and results from the first test day milk as predictors of disease, fertility, yield, and culling in commercial dairy herds. J. Dairy Sci. 82:295-304.

Hocquette, J. F., S. Tesseraud, I. Cassar-Malek, Y. Chilliard, and I. Ortigues-Marty. 2007. Responses to nutrients in farm animals: implications for production and quality. Animal. 1:1297-1313.

Holtenius, P., and K. Holtenius. 2007. A model to estimate insulin sensitivity in dairy cows. Acta Vet. Scand. 49:29-31.

Hove, K. 1978. Insulin secretion in lactating cows: responses to glucose infused intravenously in normal, ketonemic and starved animals. J. Dairy Sci. 61:1407-1413.

Ingvartsen, K. L., and J. B. Andersen. 2000. Integration of metabolism and intake regulation: a review focusing on periparturient animals. J. Dairy Sci. 83:1573-1597.

Ingvartsen, K. L., R. J. Dewhurst, and N. C. Friggens. 2003. On the relationship between lactational performance and health: is it yield or metabolic imbalance that cause production diseases in dairy cattle? A position paper. Livest. Prod. Sci. 83:277-308.

Jorritsma, R., T. Wensing, T. A. M. Kruip, P. L. A. M. Vos, and J. P. T. M. Noordhuizen. 2003. Metabolic changes in early lactation and impaired reproductive performance in dairy cows. Vet. Res. 34:11-26.

Kay, J. K., W. J. Weber, C. E. Moore, D. E. Bauman, L. B. Hansen, H. Chester-Jones, B. A. Crooker, and L. H. Baumgard. 2005. Effects of week of lactation and genetic selection for milk yield on milk fatty acid composition in Holstein cows. J. Dairy Sci. 88:3886-3893.

Kelley, K. M., Y. Oh, S. E. Gargosky, Z. Gucev, T. Matsumoto, V. Hwa, L. Ng, D. M. Simpson, and R. G. Rosenfeld. 1996. Insulin-like growth factor-binding proteins (IGFBPs) and their regulatory dynamics. Int. J. Biochem. Cell Biol. 28:619-637.

Kerestes, M., V. Faigl, M. Kulcsár, O. Balogh, J. Foeldi, H. Fébel, Y. Chilliard, and G. Huszenicza. 2009. Periparturient insulin secretion and whole-body insulin responsiveness in dairy cows showing various forms of ketone pattern with or without puerperal metritis. Domest. Anim. Endocrinol. 37:250-261.

Kessel., S., M. Stroehl, H. H. D. Meyer, S. Hiss, H. Sauerwein, F. J. Schwarz, and R. M. Bruckmaier. 2008. Individual variability in physiological adaptation to metabolic stress during early lactation in dairy cows kept under equal conditions. J. Anim. Sci. 86:2903-2912.

Kim, J. W., R. P. Rhoads, S. S. Block, T. R. Overton, S. J. Frank, and Y. R. Boisclair. 2004. Dairy cows experience selective reduction of the hepatic growth hormone receptor during the periparturient period. J. Endocrinol. 181:281-290.

Knight, C. H., D. E. Beever, and A. Sorensen. 1999. Metabolic loads to be expected from different genotypes under different systems. Metabolic stress in dairy cows. British Society of Animal Science. Occasional Publication No. 24, 27–36.

Kobayashi, Y., C. K. Boyd, C. J. Bracken, W. R. Lamberson, D. H. Keisler, and M. C. Lucy. 1999. Reduced growth hormone receptor (GHR) messenger RNA in liver of periparturient cattle is caused by a specific down-regulation of GHR 1A that is associated with decreased insulin-like growth factor-I. Endocrinology. 140:3947-3954.

Kobayashi, Y., C. K. Boyd, B. L. McCormack, and M C. Lucy. 2002. Reduced insulin-like growth factor-I after acute feed restriction in lactating dairy cows is independent of changes in growth hormone receptor 1A mRNA. J. Dairy Sci. 85:748-754.

Kreuzer, M., M. Kirchgessner, and J. W. Blum. 1991. Concentrations of hormones and metabolites in blood plasma of cows during and subsequent to different crude protein supply. J. Anim. Physiol. Anim. Nutr. 65:11-20.

Kristensen, N. B., G. Gäbel, S. G. Pierzynowski, and A. Danfaer. 2000. Portal recovery of short-chain fatty acids infused into the temporarily-isolated and washed reticulo-rumen of sheep. Br. J. Nutr. 84:477-482.

Leiber, F., M. Kreuzer, D. Nigg, H.-R. Wettstein, and M. R. L. Scheeder. 2005. A study on the causes for the elevated n-3 fatty acids in cows' milk of alpine origin. Lipids. 40:191-202.

Liefers, S. C., R. F. Veerkamp, M. F. W. te Pas, C. Delavaud, Y. Chilliard, and T. van der Lende. 2003. Leptin concentrations in relation to energy balance, milk yield, intake, live weight, and estrus in dairy cows. J. Dairy Sci. 86:799-807.

Livak, K. J., and T. D. Schmittgen. 2001. Analysis of relative gene expression data using real-time quantitative PCR and the $2^{-\Delta\Delta CT}$ method. Methods. 25:402-408.

Lopez, H., L. D. Satter, and M. C. Wiltbank. 2004. Relationship between level of milk production and estrous behavior of lactating dairy cows. Anim. Reprod. Sci. 81:209-223.

Lucy, M. C., H. Jiang, and Y. Kobayashi. 2001. Changes in the somatotropic axis associated with the initiation of lactation. J. Dairy Sci. 84(E Suppl.):E113-E119.

Luick, J. R., and L. M. Smith. 1963. Fatty acid synthesis during fasting and bovine ketosis. J. Dairy Sci. 46:1251-1255.

McCarthy, S. D., S. T. Butler, J. Patton, M. Daly, D. G. Morris, D. A. Kenny, and S. M. Waters. 2009. Differences in the expression of genes involved in the somatotropic axis in divergent strains of Holstein-Friesian dairy cows during early and mid lactation. J. Dairy Sci. 92:5229-5238.

Meier, S., P. J. S. Gore, C. M. E. Barnett, R. T. Cursons, D. E. Phipps, K. A. Watkins, and G. A. Verkerk. 2008. Metabolic adaptations associated with irreversible glucose loss are different to those observed during under-nutrition. Domest. Anim. Endocrinol. 34:269-277.

Moate, P.J., W. Chalupa, R. C. Boston, and I. J. Lean. 2007. Milk fatty acids. I. Variation in the concentration of individual fatty acids in bovine milk. J. Dairy Sci. 90:4730-4739.

Morrill, J. L., A. D. Dayton, and K. C. Behnke. 1981. Increasing consumption of dry feed by young calves. J. Dairy Sci. 64:2216-2219.

Naumann, K., R. Bassler, R. Seibold, and C. Barth. 2000. Die chemische Untersuchung von Futtermitteln, Methodenbuch Bd. III. [The chemical analysis of feedstuffs. Book of methods no. III]. Verband Deutscher Landwirtschaftlicher Untersuchungs- und Forschungsanstalten. VDLUFA-Press, Darmstadt, Germany.

NRC (National Research Council). 2001. Nutrient requirements of dairy cattle. Seventh revised edition. National Academic Press, Washington, D. C.

Ohtsuka, H., M. Koiwa, A. Hatsugaya, K. Kudo, F. Hoshi, N. Itoh, H. Yokota, H. Okada, and S. Kawamura. 2001. Relationship between serum tumor necrosis factor-alpha activity and insulin resistance in dairy cows affected with naturally occurring fatty liver. J. Vet. Med. Sci. 63:1021-1025.

Orlowski, C. C., A. L. Brown, G. T. Ooi, Y. W.-H. Yang, L. Y.-H. Tseng, and M. M. Rechler. 1990. Tissue developmental, and metabolic regulation of messenger ribonucleic acid encoding a rat insulin-like growth factor-binding protein. Endocrinology. 126:644-652.

Palmquist, D. L., A. D. Beaulieu, and D. M. Barbano. 1993. ADSA foundation symposium: Milk fat synthesis and modification. Feed and animal factors influencing milk fat composition. J. Dairy Sci. 76:1753-1771.

Perseghin, G., A. Caumo, M. Caloni, G. Testolin, and L. Luzi. 2001. Incorporation of the fasting plasma FFA concentration into QUICKI improves its association with insulin sensitivity in non-obese individuals. J. Clin. Endocrinol. Metab. 86:4776-4781.

Pezzi, C., P. A. Accorsi, D. Vigo, N. Govoni, and R. Gaiani. 2003. 5´-Deiodinase activity and circulating thyronines in lactating cows. J. Dairy Sci. 86:152-158.

Piepenbrink, M. S., A. L. Marr, M. R. Waldron, W. R. Butler, T. R. Overton, M. Vázquez-Anón, and M. D. Holt. 2004. Feeding 2-hydroxy-4-(methylthio)-butanoic acid to periparturient dairy cows improves milk production but not hepatic metabolism. J. Dairy Sci. 87:1071-1084.

Radcliff, R. P., B. L. McCormack, B. A. Crooker, and M. C. Lucy. 2003. Plasma hormones and expression of growth hormone receptor and insulin-like growth factor-I mRNA in hepatic tissue of periparturient dairy cows. J. Dairy Sci. 86:3920-3926.

Radcliff, R. P., B. L. McCormack, D. H. Keisler, B. A. Crooker, and M. C. Lucy. 2006. Partial feed restriction decreases growth hormone receptor 1A mRNA expression in postpartum dairy cows. J. Dairy Sci. 89:611-619.

Reist, M., D. Erdin, D. von Euw, K. Tschuemperlin, H. Leuenberger, C. Delavaud, Y. Chilliard, H. M. Hammon, N. Kuenzi, and J. W. Blum. 2003. Concentrate feeding strategy in lactating dairy cow: Metabolic and endocrine changes with emphasis on leptin. J. Dairy Sci. 86:1690-1706.

Renaville, R., M. Hammadi, and D. Portetelle. 2002. Role of somatotropic axis in the mammalian metabolism. Domest. Anim. Endocrinol. 23:351-360.

Rhoads, R. P., J. W. Kim, B. J. Leury, L. H. Baumgard, N. Segoale, S. J. Frank, D. E. Bauman, and Y. R. Boisclair. 2004. Insulin increases the abundance of the growth hormone receptor in liver and adipose tissue of periparturient dairy cows. J. Nutr. 134:1020-1027.

Rhoads, M. L., J. P. Meyer, W. R. Lamberson, D. H. Keisler, and M. C. Lucy. 2008. Uterine and hepatic gene expression in relation to days postpartum, estrus, and pregnancy in postpartum dairy cows. J. Dairy Sci. 91:140-150.

Röhrmoser, G., and M. Kirchgessner. 1982. Milk yield and milk ingredients of cows with undersupply in energy followed by realimentation. Züchtungskunde. 54:276-287.

Ronge, H., and J. W. Blum. 1989. Insulinlike growthfactor I responses to growth hormone in dry and lactating dairy cows. J. Anim. Physiol. Anim. Nutr. 62:280-288.

Ronge, H., J. Blum, C. Clement, F. Jans, H. Leuenberger, and H. Binder. 1988. Somatomedin C in dairy cows related to energy and protein supply and to milk production. Anim. Prod. 47:165-183.

Rukkwamsuk, T., M. J. H. Geelen, T. A. M. Kruip, and T. Wensing. 2000. Interrelation of fatty acid composition in adipose tissue, serum, and liver of dairy cows during the development of fatty liver postpartum. J. Dairy Sci. 83:52-59.

Sauerwein, H., U. Heintges, M. Hennies, T. Selhorst, and A. Daxenberger. 2004. Growth hormone induced alterations of leptin serum concentrations in dairy cows as measured by a novel enzyme immunoassay. Livest. Prod. Sci. 87:189-195.

Schröder, U. J., and R. Staufenbiel. 2006. Invited review: Methods to determine body fat reserves in the dairy cow with special regard to ultrasonographic measurement of backfat thickness. J. Dairy Sci. 89:1-14.

Stengärde, L., K. Holtenius, M. Tråvén, J. Hultgren, R. Niskanen, and U. Emanuelson. 2010. Blood profiles in dairy cows with displaced abomasum. J. Dairy Sci. 93:4691-4699.

Stoop, W. M., H. Bovenhuis, J. M. L. Heck, and J. A. M. van Arendonk. 2009. Effect of lactation stage and energy status on milk fat composition of Holstein-Friesian cows. J. Dairy Sci. 92:1469-1478.

Stull, J. W., W. H. Brown, C. Valdez, and H. Tucker. 1966. Fatty acid composition of milk. III. Variation with stage of lactation. J. Dairy Sci. 49:1401-1405.

Thissen, J. P., J. M. Ketelslegers, and L. E. Underwood. 1994. Nutritional regulation of the insulin-like growth factors. Endocr. Rev. 15:80-101.

Trigg, T. E., K. E. Jury, A. M. Bryant, and C. R. Parr. 1979. The energy metabolism of dairy cows underfed in early lactation. In: Energy Metabolism, EAAP publication No. 26, 1979, Proceedings of the Eighth Symposium on Energy Metabolism, Cambridge, UK, September 1979 (ed. L. E. Mount), 345-349.

Vandehaar, M. J., B. K. Sharma, and R. L. Fogwell. 1995. Effect of dietary energy restriction on the expression of insulin-like growth factor-I in liver and corpus luteum of heifers. J. Dairy Sci. 78:832-841.

van Dorland, H. A., S. Richter, I. Morel, M. G. Doherr, N. Castro, and R. M. Bruckmaier. 2009. Variation in hepatic regulation of metabolism during the dry period and in early lactation in dairy cows. J. Dairy Sci. 92:1924-1940.

van Haelst, Y. N. T., A. Beeckman, A. T. M van Knegsel, and V. Fievez. 2008. Short communication: Elevated concentrations of oleic acid and long-chain fatty acids in milk fat of multiparous subclinical ketotic cows. J. Dairy Sci. 91:4683-4686.

van Knegsel, A. T. M., H. van den Brand, J. Dijkstra, S. Tamminga, and B Kemp. 2005. Effect of dietary energy source on energy balance, production, metabolic disorders and reproduction in lactating dairy cattle. Review. Reprod. Nutr. Develop. 45:665-688.

van Knegsel, A. T. M. 2007. Energy partitioning in dairy cows: effects of lipogenic and glucogenic diets on energy balance, metabolites and reproduction variables in early lactation. PhD thesis. Dissertation no. 4262, Wageningen University, the Netherlands.

Veerkamp, R. F., J. K. Oldenbroek, H. J. van der Gaast, and J. H. J. van der Werf. 2000. Genetic correlation between days until start of luteal activity and milk yield, energy balance, and live weights. J. Dairy Sci. 83:577-583.

Velez, J. C., and S. S. Donkin. 2005. Feed restriction induces pyruvate carboxylase but not phosphoenolpyruvate carboxykinase in dairy cows. J. Dairy Sci. 88:2938-2948.

Vernon, R. G., R. G. P. Denis, A. Sorensen, and G. Williams. 2002. Leptin and the adaptations of lactation in rodents and ruminants. Horm. Metab. Res. 34:678-685.

Vernon, R. G., and C. M. Pond. 1997. Adaptations of maternal adipose tissue to lactation. J. Mammary Gland Biol. Neopl. 2:231-241.

Vicari, T., J. J. G. C. van den Borne, W. J. J. Gerrits, Y. Zbinden, and J. W. Blum. 2008. Postprandial blood hormone and metabolite concentrations influenced by feeding frequency and feeding level in veal calves. Domest. Anim. Endocrinol. 34:74-88.

Vicini, J. L., F. C. Buonomo, J. J. Veenhuizen, M. A. Miller, D. R. Clemmons, and R. J. Collier. 1991. Nutrient balance and stage of lactation affectresponses of insulin, insulin-like growth factors I and II, and insulin-like growth factor-binding protein 2 to somatotropin administration in dairy cows. J. Nutr. 121:1656-1664.

Wook Kim, J., R. P. Rhoads, S. S. Block, T. R. Overton, S. J. Frank, and Y. R. Boisclair. 2004. Dairy cows experience selective reduction of the hepatic growth hormone receptor during the periparturient period. J. Endocrinol. 181:281-290.

Windisch, W., M. Kirchgessner, and J. W. Blum. 1991. Hormones and metabolites in blood plasma of lactating dairy cows during and after energy and protein deficiency. J. Anim. Physiol. Anim. Nutr. 65:21-27.

Zhao, F. Q., W. M. Moseley, H. A. Tucker, and J. J. Kennelly. 1996. Regulation of glucose transporter gene expression in mammary gland, muscle, and fat of lactating cows by administration of bovine growth hormone and bovine growth hormone-releasing factor. J. Anim. Sci. 74:183-189.

References

6. Acknowledgements

At first I want to thank Prof. Dr. Frieder J. Schwarz and Prof. Dr. Rupert M. Bruckmaier, who made this thesis possible.

I thank Prof. Dr. Schwarz for his willingness to supervise this thesis and giving the great employment opportunities at the Institute for Animal Nutrition and at the Agricultural Research Unit Hirschau. Throughout my time studying and working at the institute he taught me to develop scientific thinking and research skills. His generous time he spent with me discussing and giving guidance is gratefully acknowledged. I want to thank him especially for encouraging me to attend national and international conferences as well as giving the chance to develop personality beyond professional background.

Special thanks to Prof. Dr. Bruckmaier, who enabled this collaborative project and gave me the opportunity to work in the laboratories of the Veterinary Physiology group, University of Bern. I thank him especially for many discussions, developing scientific approaches and writing publications.

Many thanks to Dr. Anette van Dorland for solving and creating statistical problems, her assistance in the laboratory and unfailing efforts for the papers published.

I thank Prof. Dr. Wilhelm M. Windisch for the participation in my rigorosum committee as well as Prof. Dr. Dr. Heinrich H. D. Meyer for reviewing this thesis and mentoring me during my doctoral study.

Many thanks to the director of the Agricultural Experimental Units, Dr. Harald Amon, for enabling the animal trial and the financial support of my doctoral study. Further on, the support of Dr. Arne Schieder and the Faculty Graduate Center Weihenstephan of the TUM-Graduate School is gratefully acknowledged.

I extend my thanks to all colleagues, fellow PhD students and employees of the Agricultural Experimental Unit Hirschau, of the Chair of Animal Nutrition and of the Veterinary Physiology group.

Last but not least, many thanks to my family for their support during my study.

Acknowledgements

7. Overview scientific communications

Peer reviewed original papers

Gross, J., H.A. van Dorland, F. J. Schwarz, R.M. Bruckmaier (2011): Endocrine changes and liver mRNA abundance of somatotropic axis and insulin system constituents during negative energy balance at different stages of lactation in dairy cows. J. Dairy Sci. doi:10.3168/jds.2011-4251 (accepted).

Gross, J., H.A. van Dorland, R.M. Bruckmaier, F. J. Schwarz (2011): Performance and metabolic profile of dairy cows during a lactational and deliberately induced negative energy balance by feed restriction with subsequent realimentation. J. Dairy Sci. 94(4): 1820-1830.

Contributions to scientific conferences

2008:

Groß, J., Sami, A.S., Schuster, M., Schwarz, F.J.: Untersuchungen zum Einsatz von Sojaextraktionsschrot, Rapsextraktionsschrot und Lupinen bei Mastbullen. - In: 120. VDLUFA-Kongress, Jena, 16.-19.09.2008. VDLUFA-Verlag, Darmstadt, 2008, S. 214-220 (64).

Wolf, E., Arnold, G.J., Bauersachs, S., Blum, H., Bruckmaier, R., Einspanier, R., Groß, J., Habermann, F.A., Hammon, H., Kliem, H., Reichenbach, H.-D., Schwarz, F., Sinowatz, F., von Dorland, A., Wiedemann, S., Zimmer, R., Kanitz, W.: REMEDY: Wie hängen Stoffwechselstörungen und Fruchtbarkeitsprobleme bei der Milchkuh zusammen? GENOMXPRESS 3.08 (2008) 6-7.

Schwarz, F.J., Groß, J.: Optimizing of the feed value of maize products and their feeding to dairy cows. In: Problemy agrotechniki oraz wykorzystania kukurydzy i sorgo, Poznan, 2008. Hrsg.: Uniwersytet Przyrodniczy w Poznaniu, Wydawnictwo, 181-184, 2008.

Groß, J., Sami, A. S., Schwarz, F. J.: Untersuchungen zum Einsatz von Lupinen, Rapsextraktionsschrot und Sojaextraktionsschrot bei Mastbullen. Tagung des Ausschusses Futterkonservierung und Fütterung. 12. und 13. März 2008. Futterkamp.

2009:

Liermann, T., Groß, J., Möckel, P., Pfeiffer A.-M., Jahreis, G., Schwarz, F. J. (2009) Performance, metabolic parameters and fatty acid composition of milk fat due to dietary CLA and rumen-protected fat of dairy cows. In: Ruminant Physiology, Digestion, metabolism and effects of nutrition on reproduction and welfare. Proceedings of the XIth International Symposium on Ruminant Physiology, Clermont-Ferrand, France, September 6-9 2009. (edited by: Y. Chilliard, F. Glasser, Y. Faulconnier, F. Bocquier, I. Veissier and M. Doreau), 570-571.

2010

Gross, J., H. A. van Dorland, Bruckmaier, R. M., Schwarz, F. J. (2010): Comparison of a lactational and nutrition-induced energy deficiency in high-yielding dairy cows with regard to performance and metabolism. XXVI World Buiatrics Congress, Santiago, Chile, November 14-18, 2010.

Ertl. J., **Groß, J.**, Schwarz, F. J. (2010). Mais- oder grassilagebasierte Rationen in der frühen Trockenstehzeit und ihre Auswirkungen auf Ca-, P- und Mg-Plasmagehalte trockenstehender und frischlaktierender Milchkühe. - In: 122. VDLUFA-Kongress, Kiel, 21.-24.09.2010.

Schwarz, F. J., **Groß, J.**, Hartl, C. (2010). Rationszusammensetzung und Milchqualität. - In: 122. VDLUFA-Kongress, Kiel, 21.-24.09.2010.

Groß, J., H. A. van Dorland, R. M. Bruckmaier, and F. J. Schwarz (2010). Performance and metabolism during physiological energy deficiency in early lactation and during energy restriction at 100 DIM in high-yielding dairy cows In: Energy and protein metabolism and nutrition, EAAP publication No. 127, 2010, 3rd EAAP ISEP, Parma, Italy, 6-10 September 2010 (ed. G. Matteo Corvetto), 305-306.

Groß, J., van Dorland, H.A., Bruckmaier, R.M., Schwarz, F.J.: Performance parameters of high-yielding dairy cows during early lactation, during an energy restriction at 100 DIM, and a following realimentation. - In: Proc. Soc. Nutr. Physiol., Göttingen, 09.-11.03.2010. Ed.: Gesellschaft für Ernährungsphysiologie. Frankfurt: DLG-Verlags-GmbH, 2010, p. 55 (19).

2011

Groß, J., Schwarz, F.J., van Dorland, H.A., Bruckmaier, R.M. (2011): Endocrine profile and hepatic gene expression in dairy cows during a negative energy balance in early lactation and during an energy-restriction at 100 days in milk (DIM). - In: Proc. Soc. Nutr. Physiol., Göttingen, 15.-17.03.2011. Ed.: Gesellschaft für Ernährungsphysiologie. Frankfurt: DLG-Verlags-GmbH, 2011, p. 34 (20).

J. **Gross**, H.A. van Dorland, F.J. Schwarz und R.M. Bruckmaier: Hormonprofile und die Genexpression von Faktoren der somatotropen Achse in der Leber bei negativer Energiebilanz von Kühen zu zwei Laktationszeitpunkten. In: Zukunftsträchtige Futtermittel und Zusatzstoffe, ETH-Schriftenreihe zur Tierernährung, Band 34 (Hrsg.: M. Kreuzer, T. Lanzini, M. Wanner, R. Bruckmaier, D. Guidon), Mai 2011, S. 37-40.

8. Appendix

Appendix I

Performance and metabolic profile of dairy cows during a lactational and deliberately induced negative energy balance by feed restriction with subsequent realimentation.

Journal of Dairy Science, Volume 94, No. 4, pages 1820-1830, doi:10.3168/jds.2010-3707

Gross, J., H.A. van Dorland, R.M. Bruckmaier, and F. J. Schwarz

Appendix II

Endocrine changes and liver mRNA abundance of somatotropic axis and insulin system constituents during negative energy balance at different stages of lactation in dairy cows.

Journal of Dairy Science, Volume 94, No. 7, pages 3484-3494, doi:10.3168/jds.2011-4251

Gross, J., H.A. van Dorland, F. J. Schwarz, and R.M. Bruckmaier

Appendix III

Milk fatty acid profile related to energy balance in dairy cows.

Journal of Dairy Research, Volume 78, pages 479-488, doi:10.1017/S0022029911000550

Gross, J., H.A. van Dorland, R.M. Bruckmaier, and F. J. Schwarz

Appendix I

Performance and metabolic profile of dairy cows during a lactational and deliberately induced negative energy balance by feed restriction with subsequent realimentation.

Journal of Dairy Science, Volume 94, No. 4, pages 1820-1830, doi:10.3168/jds.2010-3707

Gross, J., H.A. van Dorland, R.M. Bruckmaier, and F. J. Schwarz

Performance and metabolic profile of dairy cows during a lactational and deliberately induced negative energy balance with subsequent realimentation

J. Gross,* H. A. van Dorland,† R. M. Bruckmaier,† and F. J. Schwarz*[1]
*Department of Animal Sciences, Chair of Animal Nutrition, Technical University of Munich, Liesel-Beckmann-Str. 6, D-85350 Freising-Weihenstephan, Germany
†Veterinary Physiology, Vetsuisse Faculty, University of Bern, Bremgartenstr. 109a, CH-3001 Bern, Switzerland

ABSTRACT

Homeorhetic and homeostatic controls in dairy cows are essential for adapting to alterations in physiological and environmental conditions. To study the different mechanisms during adaptation processes, effects of a deliberately induced negative energy balance (NEB) by feed restriction near 100 d in milk (DIM) on performance and metabolic measures were compared with lactation energy deficiency after parturition. Fifty multiparous cows were studied in 3 periods (1 = early lactation up to 12 wk postpartum; 2 = feed restriction for 3 wk beginning at 98 ± 7 DIM with a feed-restricted and control group; and 3 = a subsequent realimentation period for the feed-restricted group for 8 wk). In period 1, despite NEB in early lactation [−42 MJ of net energy for lactation (NE_L)/d, wk 1 to 3] up to wk 9, milk yield increased from 27.5 ± 0.7 kg to a maximum of 39.5 ± 0.8 kg (wk 6). For period 2, the NEB was induced by individual limitation of feed quantity and reduction of dietary energy density. Feed-restricted cows experienced a greater NEB (−63 MJ of NE_L/d) than did cows in early lactation. Feed-restricted cows in period 2 showed only a small decline in milk yield of −3.1 ± 1.1 kg and milk protein content of −0.2 ± 0.1% compared with control cows (30.5 ± 1.1 kg and 3.8 ± 0.1%, respectively). In feed-restricted cows (period 2), plasma glucose was lower (−0.2 ± 0.0 mmol/L) and nonesterified fatty acids higher (+0.1 ± 0.1 mmol/L) compared with control cows. Compared with the NEB in period 1, the decreases in body weight due to the deliberately induced NEB (period 2) were greater (56 ± 4 vs. 23 ± 3 kg), but decreases in body condition score (0.16 ± 0.03 vs. 0.34 ± 0.04) and muscle diameter (2.0 ± 0.4 vs. 3.5 ± 0.4 mm) were lesser. The changes in metabolic measures in period 2 were marginal compared with the adjustments directly after parturition in

period 1. Despite the greater induced energy deficiency at 100 DIM than the early lactation NEB, the metabolic load experienced by the dairy cows was not as high as that observed in early lactation. The different effects of energy deficiency at the 2 stages in lactation show that metabolic problems in early lactating dairy cows are not due only to the NEB, but mainly to the specific metabolic regulation during this period.

Key words: negative energy balance, dairy cow, performance, metabolic parameter

INTRODUCTION

The onset of lactation in dairy cows is accompanied by low DMI and low energy availability, both of which slowly increase during the first week postpartum. During the same period, milk production steeply increases. Consequently, the energetic requirements of the early lactating cow are not met by her energy intake. This status is called a negative energy balance (**NEB**), and is described in most studies of newly lactating cows except those of Kessel et al. (2008) and van Dorland et al. (2009). A more adequate term that Butler et al. (2003) proposed might be "lactation-induced NEB" as this situation occurs naturally after calving and depends on the amount of milk yield and simultaneous DMI. The NEB in early lactation can be accompanied by health disorders (Bertoni et al., 2009).

Negative energy balance is associated with mobilization of body reserves, predominantly localized in fat and muscle tissue, because of homeorhetic control with highest priority for nutrient partitioning toward the mammary gland (Bauman and Currie, 1980). The priority of milk production after parturition is expressed by increased milk yield despite the physiological NEB. Plasma NEFA and ketone body concentrations increase during this early lactation stage and peak before maximum milk yield. The lactation-induced NEB may last up to 14 wk of lactation, whereas the peak of milk yield is found between wk 4 and 8 postpartum (NRC, 2001).

Received August 10, 2010.
Accepted December 22, 2010.
[1]Corresponding author: schwarzf@wzw.tum.de

An NEB may occur later in lactation during insufficient supply and quality of feed. This is seen in pastured high-yielding dairy cows and in dairy cows fed a TMR without taking into account the different performance levels and individual requirements of the cow. In this respect, energy density of the diet can be a limiting factor affecting performance. In these situations, dairy cows need to adapt to maintain homeostasis. Homeostasis is the property that regulates the internal environment and tends to maintain a stable physiological condition (Cannon, 1929; Bauman and Currie, 1980), such as the established lactation after the NEB period; that is, in mid lactation or in the so-called production phase of lactation, during which the metabolic priority of the mammary gland no longer exists. Induced NEB at this stage of lactation resulted in a decreased milk yield with elevated NEFA concentration (Carlson et al., 2006).

Performance and physiological reactions in dairy cows are influenced by homeorhetic and homeostatic control. To our knowledge, studies of homeorhetic and homeostatic control in early and mid lactation have not yet been carried out. Therefore, the objective of this study was to quantify and compare the performance and physiological reactions in dairy cows during NEB in early lactation and a deliberately induced NEB by feed restriction following early lactation. The hypothesis tested was that performance is differently affected by a marked NEB during homeorhetic and homeostatic control in dairy cows.

MATERIALS AND METHODS

Animal experiments were carried out at the Agricultural Experimental Unit Hirschau of the Technical University of Munich, Germany, and were approved by the responsible department for animal welfare affairs.

Animals

Fifty multiparous Holstein dairy cows (3.2 ± 0.2 parities, mean ± SEM) were studied from wk 1 prepartum to about wk 26 postpartum. The lactating herd was housed in a freestall barn. From 10 d before expected calving until d 5 postpartum, animals were fed individually in calving pens with straw bedding.

Period 1 was wk 1 prepartum to 12 postpartum, where all animals were treated as one group. In period 2, animals were allocated equally to either a control group (**C**, n = 25) or a restriction group (**R**, n = 25) according to the extent of NEB the cows experienced in period 1. The restriction phase (period 2) lasted for 3 wk and started at 98 ± 7 DIM. The week before feed restriction was classified as wk 0, where all cows were treated as one group. After 3 wk of feed restriction, period 3 started and lasted for 8 wk, during which R cows were (re)fed similarly to C cows (realimentation period).

Feeding Regimen

Animals in period 1 received a partial mixed ration 1 (**PMR 1**, Table 1) for ad libitum intake of basic feed (silages, hay) with separate and limited intake of concentrates. The PMR 1 was calculated to meet the demands for energy and protein of a cow (650 kg of BW) producing 21 kg of milk/d with an assumed DMI of 16 kg of DM/d. The PMR 1 was given once daily at 0930 h. Feed bins for recording individual PMR intake were connected to electronic balances. In addition to PMR 1, concentrate (**CONC**, Table 1) was fed at 1.3 kg of DM/d for the first 5 d of lactation. On d 6 postpartum, cows received 1.8 kg DM of CONC/d, which was increased up to 8.9 kg DM/d in the following 35 d. Thereafter, CONC was fed according to individual extra requirements for milk production. The CONC was offered in transponder-access feeding stations by an automatic feeding program (DeLaval Alpro, Glinde, Germany). Calculations for energy and protein supply followed the recommendations of the German Society of Nutrition Physiology (GfE, 2001).

At the start of period 2, R cows received PMR 1 with additional hay to reduce the energy content (**PMR 2**, Table 1). Furthermore, CONC was limited to 0.4 kg DM/d for all R cows during period 2. The amount of PMR 2 was limited in each week of period 2 to maintain an energy deficiency of a least 30% of the calculated requirements. Consequently, the protein supply was reduced correspondingly to obtain a stable energy:protein ratio. The C cows were maintained on PMR 1 ad libitum as in period 1. In period 3, R cows had free access to PMR 1 until the end of the study. The CONC was set from 0.4 to 4.5 kg DM/d (the mean value of the C group) in wk 1 of realimentation. During the remainder of period 3, CONC was adapted weekly for all animals as described above. For each cow, daily DMI (PMR and CONC) was recorded continuously. Changes of the diets were carried out all at once within a day. All animals had free access to fresh water.

Feed Samples and Analyses

Samples of all forages and CONC were collected weekly; samples of PMR 1 and PMR 2 were obtained twice per week. For analysis of DM, fresh feeds were weighed, dried for 24 h at 60°C, and reweighed. Sam-

Table 1. Composition and nutrient values of experimental diets and concentrate (CONC)

Item	Partial mixed ration[1]		CONC[2]
	PMR 1	PMR 2	
Components (% in DM)			
Grass silage	33.7	21.8	
Corn silage	44.9	29.1	
Hay	6.5	39.4	
Concentrate[3]	14.9	9.7	
Nutrient values			
Energy[4] (MJ of NE_L/kg of DM)	6.53	6.24	7.96
Crude fiber (g/kg of DM)	214	251	62
Crude ash (g/kg of DM)	76	75	76
Crude fat (g/kg of DM)	32	28	24
CP (g/kg of DM)	146	138	216
ADF (g/kg of DM)	254	313	84.1
NDF (g/kg of DM)	431	529	184
Lignin (g/kg of DM)	23.6	32.4	3.9
$NFC^{4,5}$ (g/kg of DM)	316	230	500
Available CP^4 (g/kg of DM)	143	137	172
Ruminal N balance[4] (g/kg of DM)	0.88	0.18	2.37

[1]PMR 1 was calculated to meet the demands for energy and protein of a cow (650 kg of BW) producing 21 kg of milk/d with an assumed DMI of 16 kg of DM/d; PMR 2 = PMR 1 with additional hay to reduce the energy content and fed to restricted cows in period 2.

[2]Additional concentrate provided according to milk yield, consisting of (% in DM) 14.9% barley, 24.8% corn kernels, 21.8% wheat, 20.1% soybean meal, 15.2% dried sugar beet pulp with molasses, and 3.2% vitamin-mineral premix including limestone.

[3]Concentrate (% in DM): 7.9% barley, 24.7% wheat, 60.0% soybean meal, 7.3% vitamin-mineral premix including salt and limestone.

[4]Calculated values.

[5]Calculated by difference: 100 − (% CP + % NDF + % crude fat + % crude ash).

ples were milled (Brabender, Duisburg, Germany; filter width 1.1 mm) and mixed into 2-wk sample pools (a 4-wk sample was pooled for CONC) for further analyses. Feed samples were analyzed for crude ash, crude fiber, and crude fat according to Weende analysis (Naumann et al., 2000). Crude protein (N × 6.25) content was determined by Dumas method, and NDF, ADF, and lignin were analyzed according to Naumann et al. (2000). Net energy (NE_L) and available CP at the duodenum (**ACP**) of the feed samples were calculated according to the German Society of Nutrition Physiology (GfE, 2001).

BW, BCS, and Ultrasonographic Measurements

Body weight was recorded automatically on electronic scales mounted in the concentrate feeders. Body condition was scored according to Edmonson et al. (1989) on a scale of 1 to 5 (1 = thin, 5 = obese). Simultaneously, B-mode ultrasonographic measurements of the longissimus dorsi muscle diameter (**MD**) and backfat thickness (**BFT**) were performed as specified in Bruckmaier et al. (1998a). The MD and BFT were evaluated graphically according to Bruckmaier et al. (1998b) using Adobe Photoshop CS4 Extended (Adobe Systems Inc., San Jose, CA). The BCS and ultrasonic measurements were performed at the same time by the same person.

Milk and Blood Samples

Cows were milked twice daily in a 2 × 6 milking parlor (DeLaval) at 0500 and 1500 h. Daily milk yield was recorded electronically. During the colostrum period or treatment of mastitis, the harvested milk was separated and manually weighed. Milk samples (about 50 mL) were collected beginning at 3 d postpartum twice weekly on 2 consecutive milkings each (Monday p.m., Tuesday a.m., Thursday p.m., and Friday a.m.). Average fat, protein, and lactose concentrations were determined by an infrared analyzer (MilkoScan FT-6000, Foss Analytical A/S, Hillerød, Denmark; Milchprüfring Bayern e.V., Wolnzach, Germany).

Blood samples were collected weekly; sampling was performed after milking before feeding between 0730 and 0900 h. Blood was collected via jugular puncture in 2 K_3EDTA-coated (18 mL) evacuated tubes (Greiner, Frickenhausen, Germany). Samples were cooled on wet ice, centrifuged at 2,000 × g for 15 min, and the plasma was aliquoted into 1.5-mL Eppendorf tubes, and stored at −20°C until analysis.

Energy and Protein Balance Calculations

Energy balance was calculated for each cow individually as the difference between energy intake through feed and energetic output for maintenance and milk production. Energy intake was determined by multiplying average weekly DMI of PMR 1, PMR 2, and CONC with the corresponding NE_L values. Maintenance requirement was quantified according to GfE (2001) by using the average weekly BW of the animal. Milk energy output resulted from milk yield and contents of mean fat, protein, and lactose of 1 wk samples according to GfE (2001). Mobilization or deposition of body tissue, in cases of negative and positive energy balance, respectively, were not accounted for in the calculations. The ACP at the duodenum (g/d) was calculated for each cow individually as the difference between protein intake through feed and protein output for maintenance and milk production according to GfE (2001).

Blood Plasma Metabolites

Concentration of glucose was measured using a kit from bioMérieux (Geneva, Switzerland; no. 61269); of NEFA with kit no. FA 115, and of BHBA with kit no. RB 1007 (both from Randox Laboratories Ltd., Schwyz, Switzerland).

Animal Health

Occurrences of diseases and health disorders, detected by daily animal inspections with veterinarian assistance, were documented and assigned to one of the following classes: mastitis and other udder-related problems, reproductive tract and related problems, claw problems, or milk fever.

Statistical Analysis

Data presented are means ± SEM. First, to evaluate the effect of the deliberately induced NEB at 100 DIM, performance and metabolic data from the control and treatment groups in period 2 and 3 were compared using the MIXED procedure of SAS (version 9.2, SAS Institute, Cary, NC). The model included week, group, lactation number, and week × group interaction as fixed effects. The area under the curve (**AUC**) of the respective measures from wk 1 to 12 postpartum was included additionally as a co-variable. The repeated subject was the individual cow. The differences between the R and C groups over time were detected by the Bonferroni t-test.

Second, the reactions of cows to the NEB in period 1 were compared with the reactions in period 2. This comparison was performed based on AUC differences/week ($\Delta AUC/wk$) calculated for each period from the cows experiencing NEB (period 1, wk 1 to 3 postpartum; period 2, R cows) and during the time they did not (period 1, wk 1 prepartum; period 2, C cows). The calculated $\Delta AUC/wk$ for the measured traits in periods 1 and 2 were statistically compared by using the MIXED procedure of SAS with period and lactation number as fixed effects and the individual cow as repeated subject. The differences between the periods were detected by the Bonferroni t-test; P-values <0.05 were considered significant.

Third, for the statistical analysis of occurrence of health disorders, a 1-sample binomial test was used to evaluate the differences between the 2 groups.

RESULTS

Feed Intake and Energy Balance

In period 1, mean total DMI (Figure 1A) increased weekly from 14.9 ± 0.2 kg/d (wk 1 postpartum) to stable values between 22 and 23 kg/d in wk 7 to 12 postpartum. The postpartum energy balance (**EB**) followed a similar pattern (Figure 1B), with the lowest values after calving (−46.1 ± 3.4 MJ of NE_L/d) and reaching positive values in wk 9 postpartum. At the beginning of lactation, cows met their energetic demands up to 70 ± 2%, whereas in wk 12 postpartum, the energy intake reached a level of 106 ± 2% of the calculated energy requirements.

In period 2, DMI for R cows decreased from 22.0 to 10.8 kg/d within 1 wk of feed restriction and stayed at 10.0 kg/d per cow in wk 2 and 3 of restriction ($P < 0.001$). The R cows experienced a NEB of −62.7 MJ of NE_L/d during the 3 wk of restriction ($P < 0.001$), and only 51 ± 2% of their energy requirements was covered.

Within the first week in period 3, C cows had a higher DMI than R cows. The EB for R cows returned to positive within wk 2 of realimentation. From wk 3 to 8, the calculated energy requirement was met by 109%, whereas C cows had a mean coverage of EB of 108%.

The mean ACP (g/d per cow) is shown in Figure 1C; it followed a similar pattern to DMI and EB and was affected by treatment in a similar manner to EB.

Milk Yield and Milk Composition

In period 1, milk yield started with 27.5 ± 0.7 kg/d (mean milk yield of d 4 to 11 postpartum), reached a peak of 39.5 ± 0.8 kg/d in wk 6 postpartum, and declined to 33.7 ± 1.1 kg/d in wk 12 postpartum (Figure 1D). Figure 2A shows the changes of milk fat and protein content. Both measures were highest in wk 1 postpartum (fat: 5.48 ± 0.12%; protein: 4.09 ± 0.06%). The fat to protein ratio (Figure 2B) in period 1 peaked at 1.51 ± 0.04 in wk 3 postpartum, and declined to relatively constant values around 1.3 from wk 7 to 12 postpartum. Milk lactose increased from 4.46 ± 0.02% in wk 1 postpartum to constant values around 4.77 ± 0.02% in wk 3 postpartum.

In period 2, R cows showed a moderate but significantly decreased milk yield (27.4 ± 0.5 kg/d) during the 3 wk of feed restriction compared with C cows (30.5 ± 0.7 kg/d; $P < 0.05$). Only in wk 1 of period 2 was there a tendency for higher milk fat percentage in R cows ($P < 0.10$) than in C cows (4.63 ± 0.15% and 4.38 ± 0.11%, respectively). During the remainder of period 2, no differences were found between the 2 groups. The fat yield calculated over the entire restriction period (Figure 2C) was lower for R cows compared with C cows (1,211 ± 22 vs. 1,335 ± 29 g/d). Furthermore, in period 2, milk protein concentration was lower ($P < 0.05$) in R cows than in C cows (3.19 ± 0.03% and 3.38 ± 0.03%, respectively, Figure 2A), and protein yield over the entire restriction period (Figure 2D) was lower in R cows during period 2 (868 ± 13 vs. 1,027 ± 22 g/d; $P < 0.001$). As a result, the R cows showed a higher mean fat to protein ratio (Figure 2B) compared with the C group in period 2 during the entire restriction period (1.40 ± 0.03 vs. 1.30 ± 0.03; $P < 0.05$).

During realimentation, in period 3, milk yield recovered and did not differ between R and C cows ($P = 0.63$). During period 3, no significant differences between the 2 groups were found for milk fat percentage. In wk 1 of period 3, R cows were lower in milk protein content compared with C cows ($P < 0.05$), and in wk 2 of period 3, a tendency ($P = 0.06$) still existed for lower protein percentage in the R cows. The fat to protein ratio in period 3 was not different between R and C cows. Feed restriction and subsequent realimentation did not affect lactose content.

BW, BCS, and Ultrasonographic Measurements

Mean BW (Figure 3A) per cow declined after parturition and remained around 650 kg from wk 7 to 12 postpartum. In the first week of feed restriction, the BW of R cows decreased and was lower than that of C cows in wk 2 and wk 3 of period 2 ($P < 0.001$). In period 3, R cows gained BW and reached a similar BW as C cows in wk 2 of realimentation. The response to NEB in BW was more intense (56 ± 4 kg) in period 2 than in period 1 (23 ± 3 kg; $P < 0.001$).

After parturition, BCS (Figure 3B) decreased to 3.05 ± 0.04 in wk 4 postpartum. In period 2, R cows showed decreasing BCS, similar to the loss of BW, that was

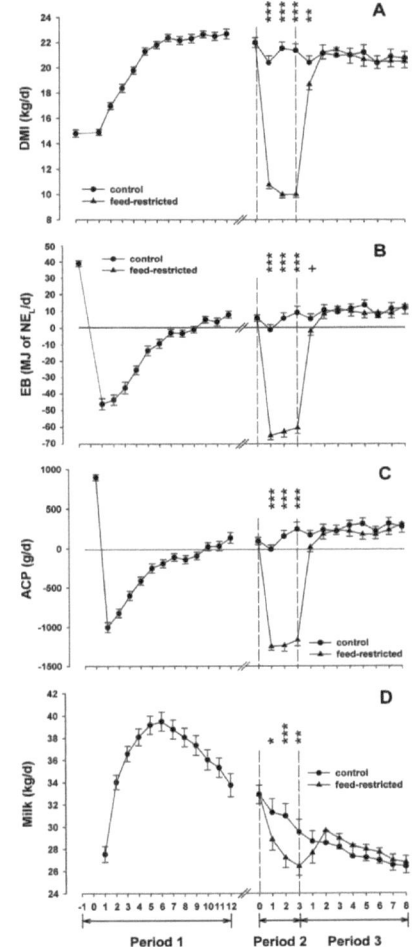

Figure 1. Dry matter intake (A), energy balance (EB; B), available CP (ACP; C), and milk yield (D) in cows during experimental period 1 (up to wk 12 postpartum), period 2 (3 wk of feed restriction), and period 3 (8 wk of realimentation). Data are given as mean values ± SEM. Differences between the groups are indicated with + ($P < 0.10$), * ($P < 0.05$), ** ($P < 0.01$), and *** ($P < 0.001$).

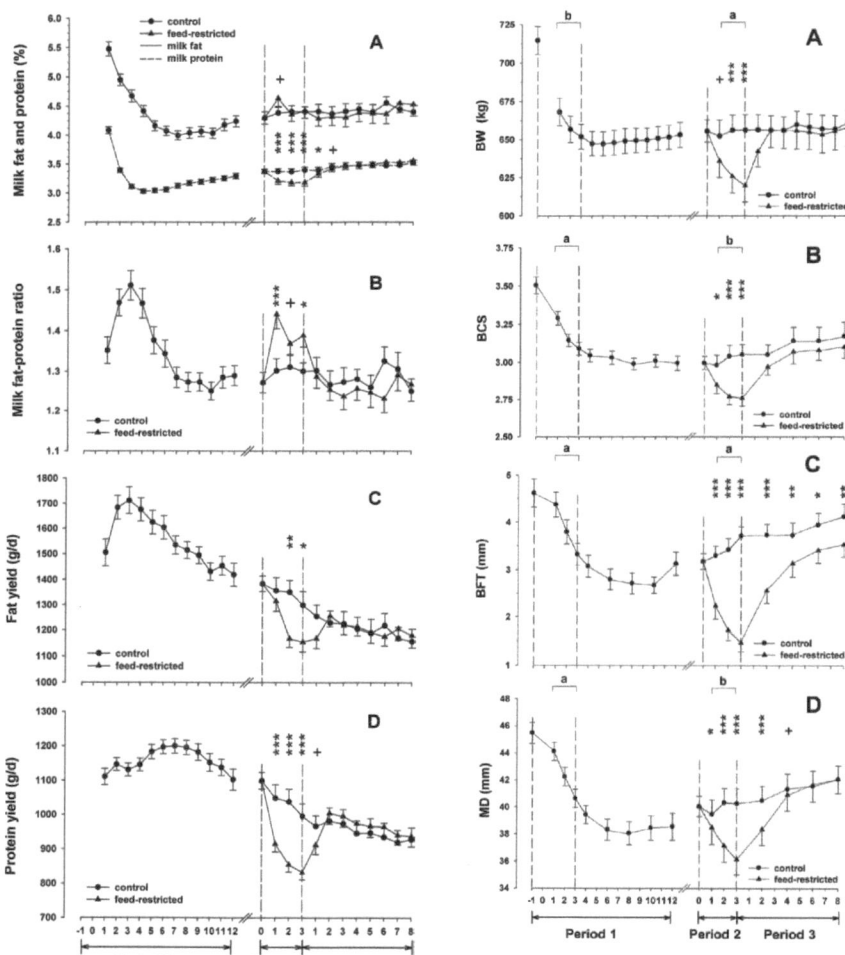

Figure 2. Milk fat and protein content (A), milk fat to protein ratio (B), fat yield (C), and protein yield (D) in cows during experimental period 1 (up to wk 12 postpartum), period 2 (3 wk of feed restriction), and period 3 (8 wk of realimentation). Data are given as mean values ± SEM. Differences between the groups are indicated with + ($P < 0.10$), * ($P < 0.05$), ** ($P < 0.01$), and *** ($P < 0.001$).

Figure 3. Body weight (A), BCS (B), backfat thickness (BFT) (C), and longissimus dorsi muscle diameter (MD) (D) in cows during experimental period 1 (up to wk 12 postpartum), period 2 (3 wk of feed restriction), and period 3 (8 wk of realimentation). Data are given as mean values ± SEM. Differences between the groups are indicated with + ($P < 0.10$), * ($P < 0.05$), ** ($P < 0.01$), and *** ($P < 0.001$). Differences between period 1 (wk 1–3 postpartum) and period 2 are indicated with different letters (a,b; $P < 0.05$).

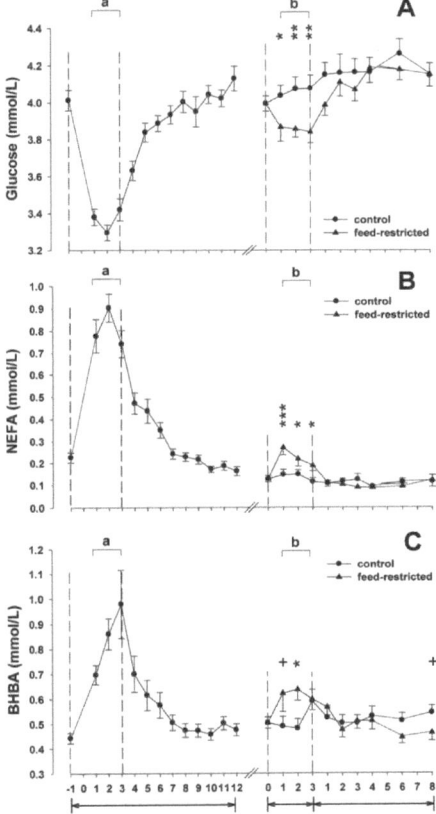

Figure 4. Concentration of plasma glucose (A), NEFA (B), and BHBA (C) in cows during experimental period 1 (up to wk 12 postpartum), period 2 (3 wk of feed restriction), and period 3 (8 wk of realimentation). Data are given as mean values ± SEM. Differences between the groups are indicated with + ($P < 0.10$), * ($P < 0.05$), ** ($P < 0.01$), and *** ($P < 0.001$). Differences between period 1 (wk 1 to 3 postpartum) and period 2 are indicated with different letters (a,b; $P < 0.05$).

lowest at the end of feed restriction ($P < 0.001$). The BCS increased in period 3 for R cows. Cows responded in BCS (Figure 3B) to NEB (Figure 1B) more intensely in period 1 (0.34 ± 0.04) than in period 2 (0.16 ± 0.03; $P < 0.01$).

The BFT (Figure 3C) was lowest in wk 10 postpartum. Within the first week of feed restriction, R cows had a rapid decline in BFT compared with C cows ($P < 0.001$). At the end of period 2, R cows had a lower BFT (3.7 ± 0.2 mm) than C cows (1.5 ± 0.2 mm; $P < 0.001$). During realimentation (period 3), BFT in R cows increased compared with C cows but did not recover during this period ($P < 0.05$). With regard to BFT, cows responded similarly to a NEB (Figure 1B) in periods 1 (0.9 ± 0.1 mm) and 2 (0.8 ± 0.1 mm; $P = 0.80$).

Similar to BFT, MD dropped from the highest value in wk 1 postpartum to the lowest values in wk 8 postpartum and remained unchanged until wk 12 postpartum (Figure 3D). In period 2, the MD of R cows decreased to wk 3 of feed restriction ($P < 0.001$). In period 3, MD increased quickly for R cows and was unchanged from wk 2 onward. The response of cows to NEB for MD was greater in period 1 than in period 2 (3.5 ± 0.4 vs. 2.0 ± 0.4 mm; $P < 0.05$).

Blood Metabolites

In period 1, plasma glucose concentrations were lowest in wk 2 postpartum (Figure 4A) and increased thereafter. Throughout period 2, mean plasma glucose concentrations were lower in R cows than in C cows (3.85 vs. 4.06 mmol/L; $P < 0.05$), and increased again in period 3 to levels similar to those of C cows. The response of cows to NEB for plasma glucose concentrations was greater during period 1 (0.65 ± 0.06 mmol/L) than during period 2 (0.16 ± 0.02 mmol/L; $P < 0.001$).

After parturition, plasma NEFA concentrations increased to wk 2 postpartum, and then decreased to wk 12 postpartum (Figure 4B). In period 2, for R cows, NEFA concentrations increased within the first week of feed restriction to 0.27 ± 0.03 mmol/L and gradually decreased thereafter. In period 3, plasma NEFA concentrations were similar for R cows and C cows. The reaction of cows to NEB for plasma NEFA concentrations was more intense in period 1 (0.59 ± 0.05 mmol/L) than in period 2 (0.08 ± 0.02 mmol/L; $P < 0.001$).

Concentrations of BHBA increased to wk 3 postpartum. Thereafter, BHBA decreased to a steady concentration of approximately 0.50 mmol/L from wk 7 to 12 postpartum (Figure 4C). During feed restriction in period 2, BHBA concentrations peaked in wk 2 at which time BHBA concentrations were higher for R cows than C cows (0.64 ± 0.04 vs. 0.48 ± 0.04 mmol/L; $P < 0.05$). In period 3, no differences between R and C cows

Table 2. Occurrence (number) of health disorders during experimental periods[1]

		Period 2			Period 3		
Health disorder	Period 1	R	C	P-value[2]	R	C	P-value[2]
Mastitis and other udder-related problems	8	0	2		4	1	
Reproductive tract-related problems	2	0	0		0	0	
Claw problems	9	2	0		0	2	
Milk fever	3	0	0		0	0	
Total	22	2	2	0.50	4	3	0.35

[1]Period 1 = wk 1 to 12 postpartum; period 2 = feed restriction for 3 wk starting at 100 DIM; period 3 = realimentation period for 8 wk after period 2. R = feed-restricted cows; C = control cows.
[2]P-values <0.05 indicate significant differences between R and C cows.

were observed for BHBA concentrations. In period 1, cows responded more intensely (0.41 ± 0.07 mmol/L) in BHBA concentrations to NEB than in period 2 (0.13 ± 0.03 mmol/L; $P < 0.01$).

Animal Health

Table 2 gives an overview of the number and type of health disorders in the different experimental periods. Based on the sum of disorders, diseases were more frequent ($P < 0.05$) in period 1 than in period 2, but R and C cows did not differ during feed restriction ($P = 0.50$) and realimentation ($P = 0.35$).

DISCUSSION

Negative energy balance can be responsible for health disorders (e.g., fertility problems, infectious diseases; Bertoni et al., 2009). On the other hand, health problems (e.g., digestive or locomotive problems) can be a trigger for NEB and may affect the NEB negatively in early lactating cows. Furthermore, the incidence of disease occurrence is closely related to high-yielding dairy cows in the transition period. This was observed in the present study, where more health problems were observed in early than in later lactation, when milk yield and metabolic stress were lower. The present study shows that metabolically more stressed cows during the NEB in early lactation simultaneously have more health disorders compared with cows experiencing a higher deliberately induced NEB with lower responses in metabolism and fewer health problems.

NEB During and Following Early Lactation

The evolution of DMI and EB after parturition in the present study followed expected patterns. After parturition, the EB decreased within a week to a nadir of −46 MJ of NE_L/d, which supports the nadir observed by Kessel et al. (2008), who conducted their study at the same research station, using the experimental herd. The total DMI supported the reports of Ingvartsen and Andersen (2000) and Kessel et al. (2008), and began at about 15 kg/d in the first week postpartum, which was higher than that reported by Ingvartsen and Andersen (2000). A plateau of DMI was reached from wk 7 postpartum onward, showing an adaptive performance of the cows, because the peak of DMI generally lags until 10 to 14 wk postpartum in early lactating dairy cows (NRC, 2001). Jorritsma et al. (2003) reported that the balance between energy from feed intake and energy requirements was attained at approximately 10 wk postpartum, which was supported by the present study, in which a positive EB was achieved in wk 9 postpartum.

The EB during the deliberately induced NEB in wk 14 postpartum decreased as suddenly as the lactation-induced NEB after parturition and achieved a nadir within 1 wk from the start of feed restriction. During the first week of the deliberately induced NEB, a NEB of −65 MJ of NE_L/d was achieved. In addition, the deliberately induced NEB remained at a level of −63 MJ of NE_L/d for 3 wk, whereas the NEB in early lactation diminished gradually after its nadir in wk 1 postpartum. This level of the deliberately induced NEB by feed restriction supported the induced NEB in other studies (Velez and Donkin, 2005; Carlson et al., 2006). The deliberately induced NEB by feed restriction was induced by reduction of DMI and energy density of the PMR. The suitability of the method was shown previously (Capuco et al., 2001).

Production Responses

From an evolutionary point of view, it is reasonable that the priority of milk production for ruminants is highest after parturition when the offspring depends on milk as the exclusive feed source (Morrill et al., 1981). The peak of milk yield was reached in wk 6 postpartum in the present study, which supports observations from the NRC (2001) and Piepenbrink et al. (2004), indicating milk production peaks between 4 and 8 wk postpartum.

Surprisingly, the decline in milk yield during the deliberately induced NEB in the present study was only about 3 kg (~10%). This was a significant decrease compared with that in the C cows, although less than the decrease of about 20% in milk yield in studies with a comparable extent of induced NEB to the present study (Velez and Donkin, 2005; Carlson et al., 2006). Among the level of the NEB induced by feed restriction, its initiation and duration must be considered in the evaluation of effects on milk production. In the present study, feed restriction lasted 3 wk starting at 100 DIM, whereas feed restriction lasted only 5 d in the study of Carlson et al. (2006), but began at 132 DIM. Furthermore, age, breed type, and genetic merit of the dairy cow may influence a cow's response to a deliberately induced energy deficiency.

During realimentation, milk yield for energy-restricted cows in the present study fully recovered to the level of the control animals. Based on calculated EB, the ad libitum feeding in this period resulted in an energy supply above cows' requirements. Besides milk yield, milk composition was affected by lactation stage and energy supply in the present study. Milk fat and protein content in early lactation decreased with the simultaneously increasing milk yield supporting Zanartu et al. (1983). During the feed restriction period in the present study, milk fat was not different in feed restriction, supporting Velez and Donkin (2005) and Carlson et al. (2006), despite a comparable NEB induced by feed restriction.

Milk protein decreased due to the energy deficiency and the simultaneous reduced protein supply during the feed restriction period. These results support studies of Röhrmoser and Kirchgessner (1982) and Carlson et al. (2006) and reflect the limited intake of feed protein. Furthermore, microbial protein synthesis in the rumen is dependent on the energy supply. Derived from milk solids, the fat to protein ratio in milk can be used as a tool indicating NEB. Heuer et al. (1999) recommend threshold values between 1.35 and 1.50, beyond which individual cows are regarded to be at higher risk for energy deficiency. When 1.35 was considered as the lower threshold, dairy cows in the present study were above this level in the first 5 wk of lactation and during the feed restriction period. The fat to protein ratio in milk partly seems a suitable instrument to detect a NEB in early and mid lactation. In contrast to milk fat and protein contents, lactose content seems to be very stable in mid and late lactation and was not affected in the present study, supporting Velez and Donkin (2005) and Carlson et al. (2006), where feed restriction did not alter milk lactose content.

Changes of BW, BCS, BFT, MD, and Blood Metabolites

In early lactation, mobilization of adipose tissue was associated with decreasing BW; it occurred simultaneously with a rapid increase of DMI. The loss of BW concomitant to the increase of DMI in early lactation was observed in a study of Liefers et al. (2003). During feed restriction, the loss of BW is a consequence of the reduced DMI and the loss of gut fill (NRC, 2001). Yet, the amount of mobilized fat can be larger than the loss of BW because the depleted body mass is partially replaced by water in the tissues (Schröder and Staufenbiel, 2006).

After a deliberately induced NEB, BW recovered in feed-restricted cows within 2 wk of realimentation, supporting Agenäs et al. (2003) who found a quick recovery of BW within 4 d of refeeding and Chelikani et al. (2004) after 24 h of refeeding after feed deprivation for 48 h. The quick increase of BW may be attributed to the increased gut fill during the refeeding period, not only to the recovery of body reserves.

To quantify the actual changes in body reserves during periods of NEB, BCS, MD, and BFT were evaluated in the present study. The BCS can mirror the nutritional status in dairy cows as it reflects changes in the subcutaneous fat layer, but BCS is influenced by subjective factors (Bruckmaier et al., 1998a). According to those authors, changes of the longissimus dorsi MD and BFT parallel those of BCS and reflect alterations of whole-body fat content and muscle mass. The decrease in BFT during the restriction period was comparable to the mobilization in early lactation (0.8 ± 0.1 vs. 0.9 ± 0.1 mm), whereas changes in MD were lower (2.0 ± 0.4 vs. 3.5 ± 0.4 mm) than in early postpartum. Furthermore, MD recovered totally in the realimentation period, whereas BFT did not recover until the end of the experiment. Björntorp et al. (1982) showed that the replenishment of lipid stores after feed restriction takes longer than refilling protein stores. The priority of body protein is maintained by limited proteolysis via endocrine control during stages of a NEB (Hocquette et al., 2007).

Plasma metabolites responded to the deliberately induced NEB at the same time as to the lactation NEB, but the extent of changes was lesser. Plasma glucose concentration decreased in the first 2 wk after parturition. According to previous studies (Baxter et al., 1956; Blum et al., 1983), this can be interpreted as a consequence of the high demand for this substrate, especially for the synthesis of lactose. The homeostatic control of blood glucose concentration in mid lactation was not affected by a partial energy restriction in the study of Carlson et al. (2006). In contrast, in the present study, plasma glucose concentration decreased during the feed restriction period. Glucose concentration was lowered by 0.2 mmol/L for feed-restricted cows (3.9 vs. 4.1 mmol/L), despite the high NEB of almost 50% of requirements. Nevertheless, energy-restricted cows after 100 DIM did not become as hypoglycemic as in early lactation.

During NEB in early lactation, body fat is mobilized and leads to increased levels of NEFA (Kessel et al., 2008; van Dorland et al., 2009). In contrast, the even greater NEB induced by feed restriction following early lactation in the present study resulted in an increase of NEFA concentration to a maximum of 0.27 mmol/L that was still below the concentration of 0.9 mmol/L observed in wk 2 postpartum. Carlson et al. (2006) found that plasma NEFA concentrations in feed-restricted cows (132 DIM) were elevated to a much lesser degree compared with the observations in early lactation.

The present study showed the highest values for BHBA during the NEB in early lactation (0.98 mmol/L in wk 3 postpartum), supporting Doepel et al. (2002) who showed that plasma BHBA concentrations peak later than NEFA concentrations. During the NEB deliberately induced by feed restriction following early lactation in the present study, R cows showed only a small change in BHBA concentration compared with control cows (0.6 vs. 0.5 mmol/L). In Carlson et al. (2006), an energy restriction of 50% did not increase BHBA concentration in feed-restricted cows. This can be explained by the smaller increase in the concentration of NEFA that serve as a substrate for ketone body production.

CONCLUSIONS

In contrast to the milk production during early lactation (Bauman and Currie, 1980), during which cows have more metabolic problems, a deliberately induced NEB at around 100 DIM resulted in an immediate but small decline of milk yield, accompanied by high losses of body reserves. In addition, the marginal changes of metabolic measures during a deliberately induced NEB by feed restriction following early lactation were within the range observed for metabolically nonchallenged cows. Therefore, the hypothesis that responses of dairy cows in performance and metabolites to a NEB in early and following early lactation are different was confirmed by the observations made in the present study. Studies on endocrine regulatory mechanisms and changes in liver metabolism designed to explain the present findings are in progress.

ACKNOWLEDGMENTS

The authors thank Yolande Zbinden (Veterinary Physiology, University of Bern) for the blood plasma analyses. The mentoring of the Graduate School (Graduate Center Weihenstephan) of the Technical University of Munich (TUM-GS) during the doctoral study of J. Gross is acknowledged.

REFERENCES

Agenäs, S., K. Dahlborn, and K. Holtenius. 2003. Changes in metabolism and milk production during and after feed deprivation in primiparous cows selected for different milk fat content. Livest. Prod. Sci. 83:153–164.

Bauman, D. E., and W. B. Currie. 1980. Partitioning of nutrients during pregnancy and lactation: A review of mechanisms involving homeostasis homeorhesis. J. Dairy Sci. 63:1514–1529.

Baxter, C. F., M. Kleiber, and A. L. Black. 1956. The blood precursors of lactose as studied with ^{14}C-labeled metabolites in intact dairy cows. Biochim. Biophys. Acta 21:277–285.

Bertoni, G., E. Trevisi, and R. Lombardelli. 2009. Some new aspects of nutrition, health conditions and fertility of intensively reared dairy cows. Ital. J. Anim. Sci. 8:491–518.

Björntorp, P., S. Edström, J. G. Kral, K. Lundholm, E. Presta, D. Walks, and M.-U. Yang. 1982. Refeeding after fasting in the rat: Energy substrate fluxes and replenishment of energy stores. Am. J. Clin. Nutr. 36:450–456.

Blum, J. W., P. Kunz, H. Leuenberger, K. Gautschi, and M. Keller. 1983. Thyroid hormones, blood plasma metabolites and haematological parameters in relationship to milk yield in dairy cows. Anim. Prod. 36:93–104.

Bruckmaier, R. M., L. Gregoretti, F. Jans, D. Faissler, and J. W. Blum. 1998a. Longissimus dorsi muscle diameter, backfat thickness, body condition scores and skinfold values related to metabolic and endocrine traits in lactating dairy cows fed crystalline fat or free fatty acids. Zentralbl. Veterinarmed. A 45:397–410.

Bruckmaier, R. M., E. Lehmann, D. Hugi, H. M. Hammon, and J. W. Blum. 1998b. Ultrasonic measurement of longissimus dorsi muscle and backfat, associated with metabolic and endocrine traits, during fattening of intact and castrated male cattle. Livest. Prod. Sci. 53:123–134.

Butler, S. T., A. L. Marr, S. H. Pelton, R. P. Radcliff, M. C. Lucy, and W. R. Butler. 2003. Insulin restores GH responsiveness during lactation-induced negative energy balance in dairy cattle: Effects on expression of IGF-I and GH receptor 1A. J. Endocrinol. 176:205–217.

Cannon, W. B. 1929. Organization for physiological homeostasis. Physiol. Rev. 9:399–431.

Capuco, A. V., D. L. Wood, T. H. Elsasser, S. Kahl, R. A. Erdman, C. P. Van Tassell, A. Lefcourt, and L. S. Piperova. 2001. Effect of somatotropin on thyroid hormones and cytokines in lactating dairy cows during ad libitum and restricted feed intake. J. Dairy Sci. 84:2430–2439.

Carlson, D. B., N. B. Litherland, H. M. Dann, J. C. Woodworth, and J. K. Drackley. 2006. Metabolic effects of abomasal L-carnitine infusion and feed restriction in lactating Holstein cows. J. Dairy Sci. 89:4819–4834.

Chelikani, P. K., J. D. Ambrose, D. H. Keisler, and J. J. Kennelly. 2004. Effect of short-term fasting on plasma concentrations of leptin and other hormones and metabolites in dairy cattle. Domest. Anim. Endocrinol. 26:33–48.

Doepel, L., H. Lapierre, and J. J. Kennelly. 2002. Peripartum performance and metabolism of dairy cows in response to prepartum energy and protein intake. J. Dairy Sci. 85:2315–2334.

Edmonson, A. J., I. J. Lean, L. D. Weaver, T. Farver, and G. Webster. 1989. A body condition scoring chart for Holstein dairy cows. J. Dairy Sci. 72:68–78.

GfE (German Society of Nutrition Physiology). 2001. Empfehlungen zur Energie- und Nährstoffversorgung der Milchkühe und Aufzuchtrinder, Ausschuss für Bedarfsnormen der Gesellschaft für Ernährungsphysiologie. DLG-Verlag, Frankfurt am Main, Germany.

Heuer, C., Y. H. Schukken, and P. Dobbelaar. 1999. Postpartum body condition score and results from the first test day milk as predictors of disease, fertility, yield, and culling in commercial dairy herds. J. Dairy Sci. 82:295–304.

Hocquette, J. F., S. Tesseraud, I. Cassar-Malek, Y. Chilliard, and I. Ortigues-Marty. 2007. Responses to nutrients in farm animals: Implications for production and quality. Animal 1:1297–1313.

Ingvartsen, K. L., and J. B. Andersen. 2000. Integration of metabolism and intake regulation: A review focusing on periparturient animals. J. Dairy Sci. 83:1573–1597.

Jorritsma, R., T. Wensing, T. A. M. Kruip, P. L. A. M. Vos, and J. P. T. M. Noordhuizen. 2003. Metabolic changes in early lactation and impaired reproductive performance in dairy cows. Vet. Res. 34:11–26.

Kessel, S., M. Stroehl, H. H. D. Meyer, S. Hiss, H. Sauerwein, F. J. Schwarz, and R. M. Bruckmaier. 2008. Individual variability in physiological adaptation to metabolic stress during early lactation in dairy cows kept under equal conditions. J. Anim. Sci. 86:2903–2912.

Liefers, S. C., R. F. Veerkamp, M. F. W. te Pas, C. Delavaud, Y. Chilliard, and T. van der Lende. 2003. Leptin concentration in relation to energy balance, milk yield, intake, live weight, and estrus in dairy cows. J. Dairy Sci. 86:799–807.

Morrill, J. L., A. D. Dayton, and K. C. Behnke. 1981. Increasing consumption of dry feed by young calves. J. Dairy Sci. 64:2216–2219.

Naumann, K., R. Bassler, R. Seibold, and C. Barth. 2000. Die chemische Untersuchung von Futtermitteln, Methodenbuch Bd. III, Verband Deutscher Landwirtschaftlicher Untersuchungs- und Forschungsanstalten. VDLUFA-Press, Darmstadt, Germany.

NRC. 2001. Nutrient Requirements of Dairy Cattle. 7th rev. ed. National Academic Press, Washington, DC.

Piepenbrink, M. S., A. L. Marr, M. R. Waldron, W. R. Butler, T. R. Overton, M. Vázquez-Anón, and M. D. Holt. 2004. Feeding 2-hydroxy-4-(methylthio)-butanoic acid to periparturient dairy cows improves milk production but not hepatic metabolism. J. Dairy Sci. 87:1071–1084.

Röhrmoser, G., and M. Kirchgessner. 1982. Milk yield and milk ingredients of cows with undersupply in energy followed by realimentation. Zuchtungskunde 54:276–287.

Schröder, U. J., and R. Staufenbiel. 2006. Invited review: Methods to determine body fat reserves in the dairy cow with special regard to ultrasonographic measurement of backfat thickness. J. Dairy Sci. 89:1–14.

van Dorland, H. A., S. Richter, I. Morel, M. G. Doherr, N. Castro, and R. M. Bruckmaier. 2009. Variation in hepatic regulation of metabolism during the dry period and in early lactation in dairy cows. J. Dairy Sci. 92:1924–1940.

Velez, J. C., and S. S. Donkin. 2005. Feed restriction induces pyruvate carboxylase but not phosphoenolpyruvate carboxykinase in dairy cows. J. Dairy Sci. 88:2938–2948.

Zanartu, D., C. E. Polan, L. E. Ferreri, and M. L. McGilliard. 1983. Effect of stage of lactation and varying available energy intake on milk production, milk composition, and subsequent tissue enzymic activity. J. Dairy Sci. 66:1644–1652.

Appendix II

Endocrine changes and liver mRNA abundance of somatotropic axis and insulin system constituents during negative energy balance at different stages of lactation in dairy cows.

Journal of Dairy Science, Volume 94, No. 7, pages 3484-3494, doi:10.3168/jds.2011-4251

Gross, J., H.A. van Dorland, F. J. Schwarz, and R.M. Bruckmaier

Endocrine changes and liver mRNA abundance of somatotropic axis and insulin system constituents during negative energy balance at different stages of lactation in dairy cows

J. Gross,* H. A. van Dorland,† F. J. Schwarz,* and R. M. Bruckmaier†[1]
*Department of Animal Sciences, Chair of Animal Nutrition, Technical University of Munich, Liesel-Beckmann-Str. 6, D-85350 Freising-Weihenstephan, Germany
†Veterinary Physiology, Vetsuisse Faculty, University of Bern, Bremgartenstr. 109a, CH-3001 Bern, Switzerland

ABSTRACT

The liver has an important role in metabolic regulation and control of the somatotropic axis to adapt successfully to physiological and environmental changes in dairy cows. The aim of this study was to investigate the adaptation to negative energy balance (NEB) at parturition and to a deliberately induced NEB by feed restriction at 100 days in milk. The hepatic gene expression and the endocrine system of the somatotropic axis and related parameters were compared between the early and late NEB period. Fifty multiparous cows were subjected to 3 periods (1 = early lactation up to 12 wk postpartum, 2 = feed restriction for 3 wk beginning at around 100 days in milk with a feed-restricted and a control group, and 3 = subsequent realimentation period for the feed-restricted group for 8 wk). In period 1, plasma growth hormone reached a maximum in early lactation, whereas insulin-like growth factor-I (IGF-I), leptin, the thyroid hormones, insulin, and the revised quantitative insulin sensitivity check index increased gradually after a nadir in early lactation. Three days after parturition, hepatic mRNA abundance of growth hormone receptor 1A, IGF-I, IGF-I receptor and IGF-binding protein-3 (IGFBP-3) were decreased, whereas mRNA of IGFBP-1 and -2 and insulin receptor were upregulated as compared with wk 3 antepartum. During period 2, feed-restricted cows showed decreased plasma concentrations of IGF-I and leptin compared with those of control cows. The revised quantitative insulin sensitivity check index was lower for feed-restricted cows (period 2) than for control cows. Compared with the NEB in period 1, the changes due to the deliberately induced NEB (period 2) in hormones were less pronounced. At the end of the 3-wk feed restriction, the mRNA abundance of IGF-I, IGFBP-1, -2, -3, and insulin receptor was increased as compared with the control group. The different effects of energy deficiency at the 2 stages in lactation show that the endocrine regulation changes qualitatively and quantitatively during the course of lactation.

Key words: negative energy balance, somatotropic axis, hormone, liver

INTRODUCTION

At the onset of lactation, nutritional and energetic requirements can increase 4-fold in high-yielding dairy cows within 1 day (Carriquiry et al., 2009). The demands for nutrients and energy cannot be met during early lactation because feed intake after parturition increases more slowly than the energetic output required by milk production. Dramatic endocrine changes occur during the transition period from late pregnancy to lactation in dairy cows to regulate the required metabolic changes.

In response to the energy deficiency, mobilization of body fat and muscle tissue occurs. The orchestrated changes in adaptation mechanisms of body tissues toward the new physiological state of priority (Bauman and Currie, 1980)—the lactation—are mediated by members of the somatotropic axis and other hormones. A pivotal role in this homeorhetic control of metabolism is played by growth hormone (**GH**), mainly mediated via IGF-I. Growth hormone directly acts on liver and adipose tissue (e.g., increases gluconeogenesis and decreases lipogenesis) as well as acting indirectly through IGF-I and IGF-binding proteins (**IGFBP**) on muscle and mammary gland (e.g., increases utilization of NEFA and increases mammary blood flow; reviewed by Renaville et al., 2002). The family of IGFBP binds circulating IGF-I and modulates its distribution and interaction with IGF-I receptors within target tissues (Renaville et al., 2002).

Simultaneously, early lactation in dairy cows is characterized by a hypoinsulinemic state. Contrary to the insulin-independent nutrient uptake in the mammary gland, low plasma insulin concentrations induce an

Received February 8, 2011.
Accepted March 13, 2011.
[1]Corresponding author: rupert.bruckmaier@vetsuisse.unibe.ch

increased oxidation of fatty acids, decreased glucose oxidation and uptake of glucose in insulin-responsive tissues (Butler et al., 2003) thus saving glucose for lactose synthesis in the mammary gland. Besides insulin and the GH-IGF-I axis, leptin (Liefers et al., 2003) and the thyroid hormones (Blum et al., 1983) play an important role in the regulation of metabolic activity during the lactational NEB and interact with other endocrine systems (Chilliard et al., 2005).

Different effects of an NEB at 2 stages in lactation (NEB in early lactation and a deliberately induced NEB by feed restriction at 100 DIM) on performance parameters and metabolites in dairy cows have been described elsewhere (Gross et al., 2011). Changes in plasma metabolites during the deliberately induced NEB were less than those occurring during the NEB in early lactation, despite the extent of the induced NEB being even higher when compared with the NEB in early lactation. In the present study, the regulation of metabolism by the somatotropic axis during these 2 periods of energy deficiency was compared and quantified based on plasma hormone concentrations and mRNA expression of related genes and receptors in the liver. The hypothesis was tested that the adaptation to NEB at parturition and to a deliberately induced NEB by feed restriction at 100 DIM is differently regulated.

MATERIALS AND METHODS

Animal Trial

The animal trial was carried out at the Agricultural Experimental Unit Hirschau of the Technical University Munich, Germany, and was approved by the state department for animal welfare affairs. The study included 50 multiparous Holstein dairy cows (3.2 ± 0.2 parities, mean ± SEM) and covered the period from wk 3 antepartum (**a.p.**) to approximately wk 26 postpartum (**p.p.**).

In experimental period 1 (wk 3 a.p. up to 12 p.p.), all cows were treated similarly. In period 2, at around 100 DIM, animals were allocated equally to either a control (**C**) or a restriction group (**R**) according to their NEB in early lactation. Each group consisted of 25 cows, and the feed restriction lasted for 3 wk. The week before feed restriction was designated as wk 0. To induce an energy deficiency of at least 30% of cow requirements at the start of period 2, R cows received a limited amount of feed from a similar diet as the C cows, but mixed with additional hay, and a decreased amount of concentrate. After 3 wk of feed restriction and established NEB, period 3 started, where R cows were (re)fed similarly as C cows for 8 wk. The feeding regimen and NEB was recently described in more detail (Gross et al., 2011).

Blood Collection and Analyses of Hormones and Metabolites

Blood samples were taken from the jugular vein between 0730 h and 0900 h before feeding in wk 3 a.p., wk 1 (on d 3), 2, 4, 8, and 12 p.p., respectively (period 1); weekly during period 2; and in wk 1, 2, 4, and 8 during period 3 and were immediately cooled down on wet ice and centrifuged for 15 min at 2,000 × g. Aliquots of EDTA blood plasma were stored at −20°C until analysis of hormones and metabolites.

Plasma GH, IGF-I, insulin, 3,5,3′-trijodthyronine (T_3) and thyroxine (T_4) were measured by radioimmunoassay as described previously Vicari et al. (2008). Plasma leptin was measured by radioimmunoassay with an antibody against bovine leptin kindly provided by Helga Sauerwein, University of Bonn, Germany (Sauerwein et al., 2004). Concentration of plasma glucose was measured using kit no. 61269 from bioMérieux (Genève, Switzerland) and of NEFA with kit no. FA 115 from Randox Laboratories Ltd. (Schwyz, Switzerland). The profiles of glucose and NEFA have been published elsewhere (Gross et al., 2011). In this paper the values are used for the calculation of the revised quantitative insulin sensitivity check index (**RQUICKI**).

As a measure of insulin sensitivity, the RQUICKI was calculated. The RQUICKI is based on the concentrations of plasma glucose, NEFA, and insulin and may be an instrument to estimate insulin sensitivity in dairy cows (Holtenius and Holtenius, 2007). The RQUICKI is estimated according to the equation given by Perseghin et al. (2001) and used by Holtenius and Holtenius (2007): RQUICKI = 1/[log(glucose) + log(insulin) + log(NEFA)].

Liver Tissue Collection, mRNA Extraction, and

Liver samples were obtained by blind percutaneous needle biopsy (14G × 152 mm; Dispomed Witt oHG, Gelnhausen, Germany) under local anesthesia after blood sampling as described by van Dorland et al. (2009) in wk 3 a.p., wk 1 p.p. (on d 3), and wk 4 p.p. (period 1), and before feed restriction in wk 0 and 3 of period 2. Liver tissue (40 to 60 mg) was put directly into an RNA stabilization reagent (RNAlater; Ambion, Applied Biosystems, Austin, TX), and kept at +4°C for 24 h, and thereafter stored at −20°C until analyzed. Total RNA was isolated from liver tissue using peqGOLD TriFast (PEQLAB Biotechnologie GmbH,

Table 1. PCR primer information, the annealing temperature, and the PCR product length for the genes analyzed in liver sample[1]

Gene[2]		Sequence 5'–3'	GeneBank accession no.	Annealing temperature (°C)	Length (bp)
GAPDH	For.	TACATGGTCTACATGTTCCAGTATG	NM 001034034	60	439
	Rev.	CAGTCTTCTGGGTGGCAGTGATG			
GHR 1A	For.	CCAGTTTCCATGGTTCTTAATTAT	NM_176608.1	60	138
	Rev.	TTCCTTTAATCTTTGGAACTGG			
IGF-I	For.	TCGCATCTCTTCTATCTGGCCCTGT	NM_001077828.1	60	240
	Rev.	GCAGTACATCTCCAGCCTCCTCAGA			
IGF-IR	For.	TTAAAATGGCCAGAACCTGAG	XM_002696504.1	60	314
	Rev.	ATTATAACCAAGCCTCCCAC			
IGFBP-1	For.	TCAAGAAGTGGAAGGAGCCCT	NM_174554.2	60	127
	Rev.	AATCCATTCTTGTTGCAGTTT			
IGFBP-2	For.	CACCGGCAGATGGGCAA	NM_174555	60	136
	Rev.	GAAGGCGCATGGTGGTGGAGAT			
IGFBP-3	For.	ACAGACACCCAGAACTTCTCCTC	NM_174556.1	60	194
	Rev.	GCTTCCTGCCCTTGGA			
INSR	For.	TCCTCAAGGAGCTGGAGGAGT	XM_002688832.1	62	163
	Rev.	GCTGCTGTCACATTCCCCA			
UBQ	For.	AGATCCAGGATAAGGAAGGCAT	Z18245	62	198
	Rev.	GCTCCACTTCCAGGGTGAT			

[1]For. = forward; Rev. = reverse.
[2]GHR 1A = growth hormone receptor 1A; IGF-IR = IGF-I receptor; IGFBP = IGF-binding protein; INSR = insulin receptor; UBQ = ubiquitin.

Erlangen, Germany) according to the manufacturer's instructions. The yield and purity of total RNA were detected by spectrophotometer with a BioPhotometer (Vaudaux-Eppendorf, Basel, Switzerland). The RNA integrity was verified by the optical density at 260 nm/280 nm (OD260/OD280) absorption ratio, which was between 1.7 and 2.1 for all samples.

For reverse transcription, 1 μg of extracted total RNA was reverse transcribed with 200 U of Moleney Murine Leukemia Virus Reverse Transcriptase RNase H Minus, Point Mutant (Promega Corp., Madison, WI) using 100 pmol of random hexamer primers (Invitrogen, Leek, the Netherlands). The obtained cDNA was diluted to a final concentration of 25 ng/μL. The genes selected to measure the expression from the somatotropic axis are described in Table 1. The PCR quantification was performed with the Rotor-Gene 6000 (Corbett Research, Sydney, Australia), using the software version 1.7.40. Fluorescence takeoff was calculated with the second derivative maximum program option. A master mix of the following reaction components was prepared: 1.8 μL of diethylpyrocarbonate (DEPC) water, 1.0 μL of forward primer (5 pmol), 1.0 μL of reverse primer (5 pmol), 0.2 μL of 50× SYBR-Green (20 pmol; Applied Biosystems), and 5.0 μL of 2× SensiMix (1 mM MgCl$_2$; 2× SensiMix NoRef DNA Kit; Bioline USA, Inc., Taunton, MA). In total, 9 μL of master-mix and 1 μL of sample volume, containing 25 ng of cDNA, were used. The following 3-step PCR program was used: denaturation for 10 min at 95°C, 40 cycles of amplification (each consisting of 15 s at 95°C, the primer specific annealing temperature for 30 s (see Table 1), and extension at 72°C for 20 s and quantification of fluorescence), and finally, a melting curve program (60 to 95°C). The mRNA abundance of target genes was calculated relative to the mRNA abundance of the reference genes GAPDH and ubiquitin (UBQ; see Table 1 for details of the primers). The mRNA levels of the housekeeping genes were stable across the time points (17.7 ± 0.1, 17.6 ± 0.2, 17.4 ± 0.2, 17.0 ± 0.1 and 17.1 ± 0.3 in wk 3 a.p., wk 1 p.p., wk 4 p.p. (period 1), and wk 0 and 3 of period 2, respectively).

Statistical Analysis

Data presented in text and figures are means ± standard error of the means. To identify changes over time within groups, data on mRNA abundance and endocrine parameters at the respective time points of liver biopsies in period 1 [wk 3 a.p., wk 1 p.p. (= d 3 p.p.), and wk 4 p.p.] and period 2 (wk 0 and 3) were evaluated by a MIXED model in SAS, version 9.2 (SAS Institute, Cary, NC) with time point and parity as fixed effects. Differences over time were detected by the Bonferroni t-test.

To evaluate the effect of feed restriction (period 2) on gene expression in liver, mRNA abundance [delta cycle threshold (CT), log$_2$] in wk 3 of period 2 was evaluated in a MIXED model including group and parity. Furthermore, the mRNA abundance of wk 0 of period 2 was used as a co-variable and individual cow as repeated subject. To evaluate effects of feed restriction on endocrine parameters for periods 2 and 3 (wk 1 to 4), the areas under the curve (**AUC**) of R and C groups were compared using the MIXED procedure of SAS. The model included group and parity as fixed effects.

The AUC from wk 8 p.p. until the beginning of period 2 (wk 0) was included additionally as a co-variable. The repeated subject was the individual cow. Group differences were detected by the Bonferroni t-test. P-values <0.05 were considered to be significant.

RESULTS

Plasma Hormones

GH, IGF-I, and Leptin. The concentration of plasma GH increased from wk 3 a.p. to a maximum in wk 1 p.p. and then gradually decreased until the start of period 2 (Figure 1A). The plasma GH concentration did not differ between wk 0 and 3 of period 2 in both groups. The AUC of GH during period 2 did not differ between groups. In addition, the GH concentration did not differ in the R group between wk 1 p.p. (period 1) and wk 3 of period 2. In period 3, the AUC of GH did not differ between the R and C group.

The plasma IGF-I concentration in period 1 decreased from a maximum in wk 3 a.p. to a nadir in wk 2 p.p. and increased steadily thereafter (Figure 1B). The plasma IGF-I concentration did not differ between wk 0 and 3 of period 2 in both groups. The AUC of IGF-I was lower in the R group than in the C group during period 2 ($P < 0.05$). The IGF-I concentration in the R group did not differ between wk 1 p.p. (period 1) and wk 3 of period 2. In period 3, the AUC of IGF-I did not differ between groups.

The leptin concentration in plasma (Figure 2A) was observed to be highest during period 1 in wk 3 a.p., reached a nadir in wk 1 p.p., and thereafter increased gradually. The plasma leptin concentration did not differ between wk 0 and 3 of period 2 for R cows. The AUC of leptin was lower in R cows compared with C cows during period 2 ($P < 0.05$). The leptin concentration did not differ between wk 1 p.p. (period 1) and wk 3 of period 2. In period 3, no differences in the AUC of leptin were found between groups.

Insulin and RQUICKI. The insulin concentration in period 1 decreased from wk 3 a.p. to a minimum in wk 1 p.p. and increased thereafter (Figure 2B). For R cows, the insulin concentration differed between wk 0 and 3 of period 2 ($P < 0.05$). The AUC of insulin did not differ between the R and C groups during period 2. The insulin concentration for R cows was different between wk 1 p.p. (period 1) and wk 3 of period 2 ($P < 0.05$). In period 3, no differences were detected for the AUC of insulin between the R and C groups.

In period 1, the RQUICKI decreased from wk 3 a.p. to a nadir in wk 2 p.p. and increased gradually thereafter (Figure 2C). Between wk 0 and 3 of period 2, the RQUICKI of R and C cows did not differ. The AUC

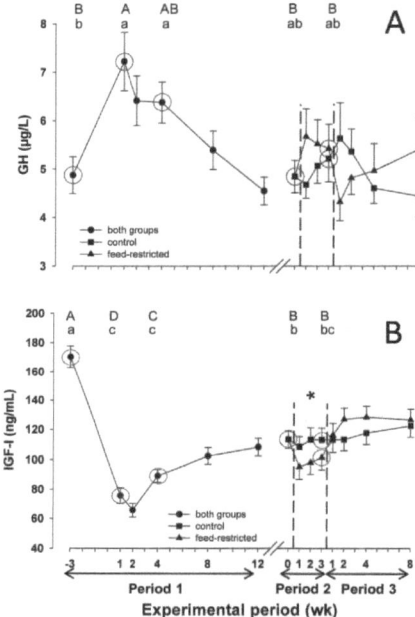

Figure 1. Plasma concentration of growth hormone (GH; A) and IGF-I (B) in cows during experimental period 1 [up to wk 12 postpartum (p.p.)], period 2 (3 wk of feed restriction), and period 3 (8 wk of realimentation). Data are given as mean values ± standard error of the means. Differences between the groups during periods 2 and 3 (wk 1 to 4) are marked with * ($P < 0.05$). Changes over time for points with simultaneous blood and liver samples (in circles) within the groups in period 1 (wk 3 antepartum, wk 1 p.p., wk 4 p.p.) and period 2 (wk 0 and 3) are marked with different letters (A–D for the control group; a–c for the feed-restricted group; $P < 0.05$).

of the RQUICKI was lower for R cows compared with C cows during period 2 ($P < 0.05$). The R cows were different in RQUICKI between wk 1 p.p. in period 1 and wk 3 of period 2 ($P < 0.05$). In period 3, the AUC of the RQUICKI did not differ between groups.

T_3, T_4, and the $T_3:T_4$ Ratio. In period 1, the plasma concentration of T_3 steadily increased from wk 3 a.p. until the beginning of period 2 (Figure 3A). For R cows, a difference in T_3 concentration between wk 0 and 3 of period 2 was observed ($P < 0.05$), whereas in C cows, the concentration did not differ. The AUC of T_3 did not differ between the R and C groups during

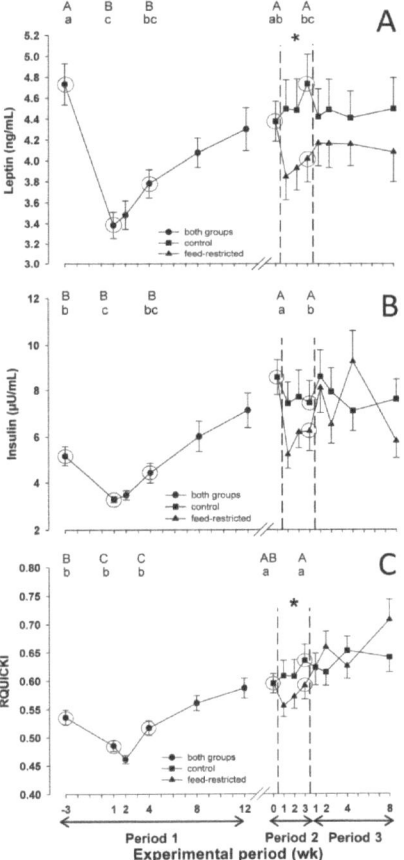

Figure 2. Plasma concentration of leptin (A), insulin (B), and the revised quantitative insulin sensitivity check index (RQUICKI; C) in cows during experimental period 1 [up to wk 12 postpartum (p.p.)], period 2 (3 wk of feed restriction), and period 3 (8 wk of realimentation). Data are given as mean values ± standard error of the means. Differences between the groups during period 2 and 3 (wk 1 to 4) are marked with * ($P < 0.05$). Changes over time for points with simultaneous blood and liver samples (in circles) within the groups in period 1 (wk 3 antepartum, wk 1 p.p., wk 4 p.p.) and period 2 (wk 0 and 3) are marked with different letters (A–C for the control group; a–c for the feed-restricted group; $P < 0.05$).

period 2. Week 1 p.p. (period 1) and wk 3 in period 2 were not different for R cows regarding plasma T_3 concentration. The AUC of T_3 during period 3 did not differ between the R and C groups.

In period 1, the plasma concentration of T_4 decreased from wk 3 a.p. to a minimum in wk 1 p.p. and increased thereafter (Figure 3B). For R cows, no difference was found between wk 0 and 3 of period 2. The AUC of T_4 did not differ between the R and C groups during period 2. The R cows differed between wk 1 p.p. (period 1) and wk 3 of period 2 in T_4 concentration ($P < 0.05$). In period 3, no difference in the AUC of the T_4 concentration was found between the groups.

In period 1, the ratio of T_3:T_4 increased from the minimum in wk 3 a.p. until wk 1 p.p. (Figure 3C) and decreased slightly thereafter. For both R and C groups, wk 0 and 3 of period 2 did not differ in the T_3:T_4-ratio. In period 2, the AUC of the T_3:T_4-ratio did not differ between the R and C groups. Between wk 1 p.p. (period 1) and wk 3 of period 2, R cows showed a difference in the T_3:T_4-ratio ($P < 0.05$). In period 3, no differences were found for the AUC of the T_3:T_4-ratio between the groups.

Changes in mRNA Abundance of Hepatic Parameters

The highest mRNA abundance of growth hormone receptor (**GHR**) 1A compared with the other time points was measured for C cows in wk 3 a.p. ($P < 0.05$), whereas R cows did not show a difference in gene expression over time (Figure 4A). In period 2, no difference was found in mRNA abundance of GHR 1A between wk 0 and 3 for the groups. In wk 3 of period 2, no differences in gene expression of GHR 1A were found between R and C groups. For R cows, expression of GHR 1A was not different between wk 1 (period 1) and wk 3 of period 2.

In wk 3 a.p. (period 1), the mRNA abundance of IGF-I was highest compared with wk 1 and 4 p.p. for both C and R groups (Figure 4B). The expression of IGF-I did not differ between wk 0 and 3 of period 2 for both groups. In wk 3 of period 2, R cows had a higher mRNA abundance than that of C cows ($P < 0.05$), which was also higher compared with wk 1 p.p. in period 1 ($P < 0.05$).

The mRNA abundance of IGF-IR was not affected over time within groups (Figure 4C). Feed restriction (wk 3 in period 2) increased the mRNA abundance of IGF-IR for R cows compared with C cows ($P < 0.05$). The gene expression of IGF-IR for R cows did not differ between wk 1 p.p. of period 1 and wk 3 of period 2.

The mRNA abundance of IGFBP-1 in period 1 increased from wk 3 a.p. to a maximum at wk 1 p.p. (Figure 5A). No differences were found for IGFBP-1 between wk 0 and 3 of period 2 for both R and C groups. The R cows showed a higher mRNA abundance of IGFBP-1 in wk 3 of period 2 compared with C cows ($P < 0.05$). The expression of IGFBP-1 for R cows was higher in wk 1 p.p. (period 1) compared with wk 3 of period 2 ($P < 0.05$).

The mRNA abundance of IGFBP-2 in period 1 increased from wk 3 a.p. to a maximum in wk 1 p.p. for C and R cows (Figure 5B) and decreased until wk 0 of period 2. Neither the R nor the C group was different in expression of IGFBP-2 between wk 0 and 3 of period 2. In wk 3 of period 2, R cows had a higher expression of IGFBP-2 than did C cows ($P < 0.05$). The IGFBP-2 concentration was different in R cows between wk 1 p.p. (period 1) and wk 3 of period 2 ($P < 0.05$).

In wk 3 a.p., the mRNA abundance of IGFBP-3 was highest (Figure 5C). The expression of IGFBP-3 was not different for R and C groups between wk 0 and 3 of period 2. The R cows had a higher mRNA abundance of IGFBP-3 in wk 3 of period 2 compared with that of C cows ($P < 0.05$). For R cows, no differences were found between wk 1 p.p. (period 1) and wk 3 of period 2.

Expression of the insulin receptor (**INSR**) in period 1 increased from wk 3 a.p. to a maximum in wk 1 p.p. and decreased thereafter (Figure 6). Between wk 0 and 3 of period 2, no differences were found in expression of the INSR for the R and C groups. In wk 3 of period 2, R cows had a higher mRNA abundance of the INSR compared with that of C cows ($P < 0.05$). For R cows, the mRNA abundance of the INSR between d 3 p.p. and wk 3 of period 2 did not differ.

DISCUSSION

The endocrine system mediates essential signals for the successful implementation and maintenance of lactation. Growth hormone and the other constituents of the somatotropic axis contribute markedly in this process during early lactation (Bauman and Currie, 1980; Bradford and Allen, 2008). The increased GH secretion during the NEB p.p. enables the shift of nutrients from body stores toward the mammary gland for milk synthesis (Bauman et al., 1982). The concentration of GH in the present study was greater during the NEB in early lactation than in the period following the NEB in agreement with Ronge et al. (1988) and Bradford and Allen (2008). A characteristic change we detected during the NEB p.p. was the downregulation of the mRNA abundance of GHR 1A, which is thought to be a key change during the uncoupling of the somatotropic axis in early lactation (Ronge et al., 1988; Lucy et al., 2001; McCarthy et al., 2009). As a consequence of uncoupling, we detected a decreased plasma IGF-I

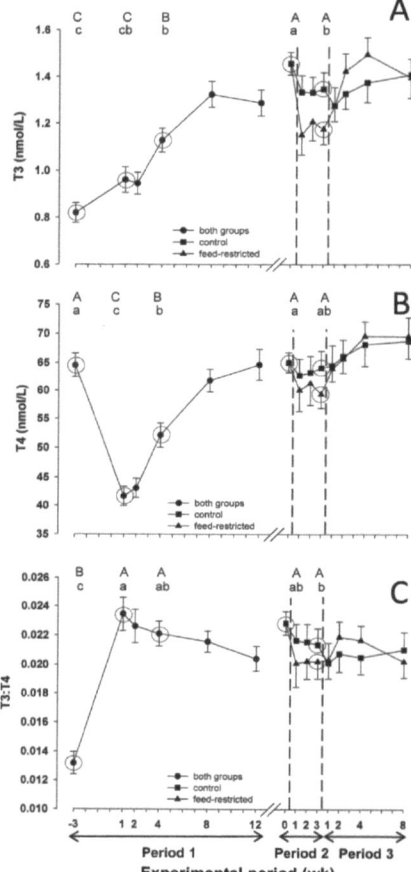

Figure 3. Plasma concentration of 3,5,3'-trijodthyronine (T_3; A), thyroxine (T_4; B), and the T_3:T_4 ratio (C) in cows during experimental period 1 [up to wk 12 postpartum (p.p.)], period 2 (3 wk of feed restriction), and period 3 (8 wk of realimentation). Data are given as mean values ± standard error of the means. Changes over time for points with simultaneous blood and liver samples (in circles) within the groups in period 1 (wk 3 antepartum, wk 1 p.p., wk 4 p.p.) and period 2 (wk 0 and 3) are marked with different letters (A–C for the control group; a–c for the feed-restricted group; $P < 0.05$).

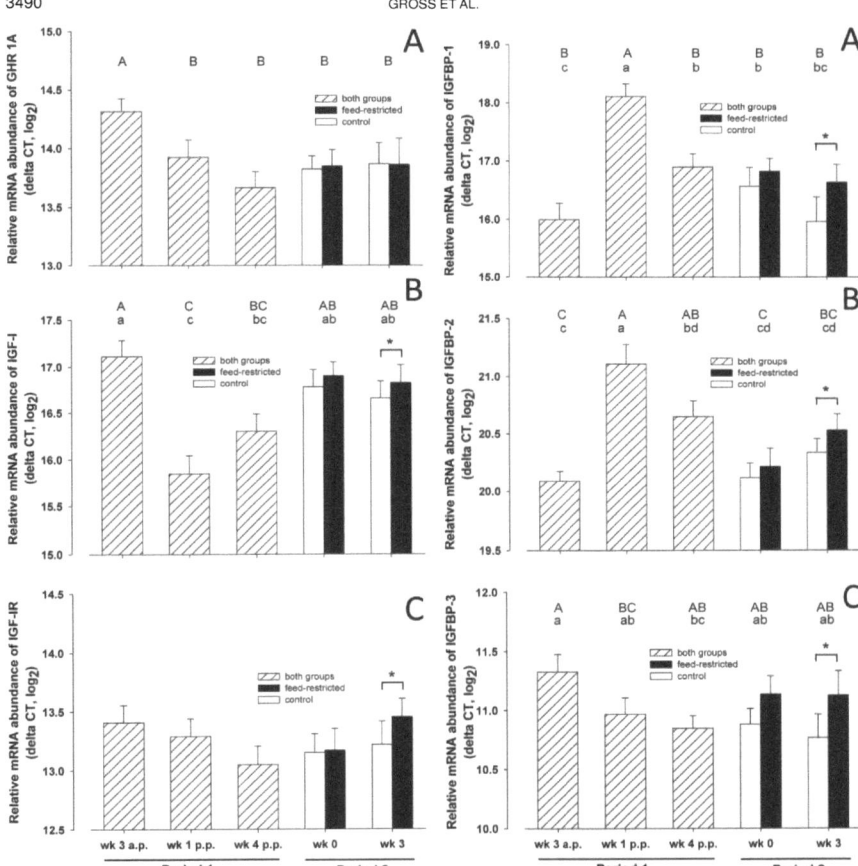

Figure 4. Relative liver mRNA abundance [delta cycle threshold (CT), $\log_2$] of growth hormone receptor (GHR 1A; A), IGF-I (B), and IGF-I receptor (IGF-IR; C) over the time points in cows during experimental period 1 [up to wk 12 postpartum (p.p.)] and period 2 (3 wk of feed restriction). Data are given as mean values ± standard error of the means. Effects of feed restriction on mRNA abundance for cows during period 2 are marked with * ($P < 0.05$). Changes over time within the groups in period 1 [wk 3 antepartum (a.p.), wk 1 p.p., wk 4 p.p.] and period 2 (wk 0 and 3) are marked with different letters (A–C for the control group; a–c for the feed-restricted group; $P < 0.05$).

Figure 5. Relative liver mRNA abundance [delta cycle threshold (CT), $\log_2$] of IGF-binding protein 1 (IGFBP-1; A), IGFBP-2 (B), and IGFBP-3 (C) over the time points in cows during experimental period 1 [up to wk 12 postpartum (p.p.)] and period 2 (3 wk of feed restriction). Data are given as mean values ± standard error of the means. Effects of feed restriction on mRNA abundance for cows during period 2 are marked with * ($P < 0.05$). Changes over time within the groups in period 1 [wk 3 antepartum (a.p.), wk 1 p.p., wk 4 p.p.] and period 2 (wk 0 and 3) are marked with different letters (A–C for the control group; a–d for the feed-restricted group; $P < 0.05$).

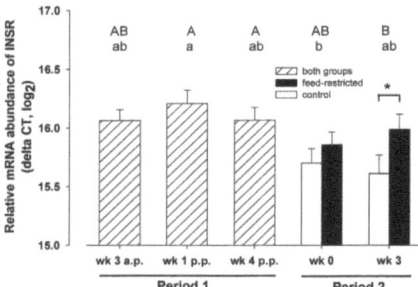

Figure 6. Relative liver mRNA abundance [delta cycle threshold (CT), $\log_2$] of insulin receptor (INSR) over the time points in cows during experimental period 1 [up to wk 12 postpartum (p.p.)] and period 2 (3 wk of feed restriction). Data are given as mean values ± standard error of the means. Effects of feed restriction on mRNA abundance for cows during period 2 are marked with * ($P < 0.05$). Changes over time within the groups in period 1 [wk 3 antepartum (a.p.), wk 1 p.p., wk 4 p.p.] and period 2 (wk 0 and 3) are marked with different letters (A, B for the control group; a, b for feed-restricted group; $P < 0.05$).

concentration from wk 3 a.p. until wk 2 p.p., which increased thereafter. These changes reflect the expected differences of hepatic IGF-I synthesis (Kobayashi et al., 1999; Butler et al., 2003; Wook Kim et al., 2004).

The decrease of plasma IGF-I also means a loss of negative feedback of GH secretion and, hence, a lack of inhibition of GH release from the pituitary and provides the explanation of high GH plasma concentrations during catabolic stages (Radcliff et al., 2006).

The responses of plasma GH and IGF-I concentration to the deliberately induced NEB were similar to the NEB p.p., but the changes were less intense. In contrast to NEB in early lactation, feed restriction did not decrease mRNA abundance of GHR 1A or of IGF-I, indicating that the endocrine adaptation to the NEB is differently mediated in these 2 periods of NEB. Other cow studies conducted later in lactation (153 to 265 DIM; Kobayashi et al., 2002) showed a decreased mRNA expression of hepatic IGF-I, but mRNA expression of GHR 1A was not changed. In still another study with feed-restricted, but nonlactating dairy cows, decreased plasma IGF-I levels were observed during the period of induced NEB and occurred concomitantly with hepatic decreasing IGF-I mRNA and GHR 1A mRNA abundance. However, no increase in plasma GH level occurred (Meier et al., 2008). These different findings illustrate a variety of different interactions between the key players of the somatotropic axis at different metabolic stages of the animal. Our results indicate a partial uncoupling of the somatotropic axis during the deliberately induced NEB as the plasma IGF-I concentration and hepatic IGF-I mRNA abundance differed between the R and C groups, whereas the plasma GH concentration was not different. The underlying partial GH resistance of the liver may be related to changes of IGFBP to induce a mechanism for the preferential utilization of mobilized substrates to maintain homeostasis rather than cell growth and proliferation in the feed-restricted animals (Renaville et al., 2002).

A higher mRNA abundance of IGFBP-1 and -2 was observed during the NEB in early lactation and deliberately induced NEB. Insulin-like growth factor-binding protein 1 gene transcription and its glucose counterregulatory role were shown to be elevated during decreased feed intake (Baxter, 1993). Because the expression of IGFBP-1 has been shown to be suppressed by both insulin and IGF-I (Kelley et al., 1996), the low levels of these factors are most likely responsible for the elevated IGFBP-1 mRNA abundance during a NEB. However, metabolic factors also may regulate IGFBP-2 in a manner similar to that of IGFBP-1. Low plasma insulin levels that occur during NEB trigger IGFBP-2 synthesis in the liver (Orlowski et al., 1990; Thissen et al., 1994). The elevation of hepatic IGFBP-2 mRNA abundance during NEB in both lactational stages is consistent with the role of IGFBP to decrease the bioavailability of IGF-I for peripheral tissues (Vicini et al., 1991; Vandehaar et al., 1995; Fenwick et al., 2008). The liver is the main contributor of IGFBP-3 in the circulation and GH is the main stimulator of IGFBP-3 (Kelley et al., 1996). Whereas the mRNA of IGFBP-3 expression was decreased during the NEB in early lactation, R cows in the present study showed a higher mRNA abundance of IGFBP-3 during the deliberately induced NEB compared with C cows. This demonstrates a difference between periods 1 and 2 in the adaptive response to NEB. Changes in IGFBP-1 and -2 during feed restriction appear to restrict the insulin-like activity of IGF-I during catabolic states, but the major decrease of IGFBP-3 likely maximizes the availability of remaining IGF-I to the tissues (Breier, 1999). According to Breier (1999), circulating IGFBP-3 and its ternary complex are decreased during periods of NEB, and the activity of an IGFBP-3-specific protease is induced to decrease IGFBP-3 affinity for IGF-I. However, during the deliberately induced NEB in the present study, the expression of IGFBP-3 did not change when compared with the beginning of feed restriction. Despite decreased circulating IGF-I in R cows, intact ternary complexes of IGF-I and IGFBP-3 appear to be changing, which may alter the interpretation of action. We report low T_3 concentrations in the dry period and early lactation, high concentrations of T_4 during the dry period, and low T_4 concentrations in early lactation. The effect of the deliberately induced NEB on thyroid hormones was less pronounced when compared with the NEB in early lactation and for period 1; the results agree with previous reports (Ronge et al., 1988; Pezzi et al., 2003). However, no significant change of T_3 and T_4 occurred during the feed restriction period as reported by Windisch et al. (1991). Thyroid gland production of T_4 is normally transformed into T_3 by 5′-deiodination in the liver, but the deiodinating system is also present in other peripheral tissues that produce T_3 according to the local requirements (Pezzi et al., 2003). The increased utilization of thyroid hormones by the mammary gland or the altered 5′-deiodinase activity in the liver are partly responsible for the hypothyroid state in early lactating animals. The hypothyroid state enhances mammary type II 5′-deiodinase and inhibits liver type I 5′-deiodinase activity (Pezzi et al., 2003). Therefore, a changed local T_3 production in the mammary gland might also be an important factor for decreased milk production during the NEB induced by feed restriction.

Plasma leptin decreased in early lactating dairy cows as well as in R cows. Block et al. (2001) attributed the postpartum decrease in plasma leptin concentration to the state of NEB caused by the initiation of lactation. Increased concentration of GH and decreased plasma insulin concentration coincide with the onset of NEB and the decrease in plasma leptin in periparturient and underfed cows (Block et al., 2001, 2003). The decrease of plasma leptin is associated with an enhanced appetite (Ingvartsen and Andersen, 2000). However, during the period of NEB postpartum, energy requirements could not be met in spite of increasing feed intake because of limited capacity of ruminal fermentation. Furthermore, leptin is partly responsible for maintaining T_4 levels (Vernon et al., 2002) and, therefore, hypoleptinemia may have been partially responsible for the hypothyroid state during periods of NEB.

The state of hypoinsulinemia in early lactating dairy cows is a major regulatory element in the adaptive system around parturition to support lactation (Butler et al., 2003). The decreased plasma insulin concentrations during the NEB in early lactation in our study decreased glucose uptake in insulin-responsive tissues (e.g., muscle and adipose tissue) and enabled more glucose uptake of the non-insulin-responsive mammary gland (Bauman and Elliot, 1983) via insulin-independent glucose transporters 1 and 3 (Zhao et al., 1996). Furthermore, insulin is hypothesized to be a key signal regulating the coupling of the somatotropic axis (Butler et al., 2003). The deliberately induced NEB study was accompanied by a protein deficiency, which would explain the rather small decrease in plasma insulin concentration compared with the decrease in early lactation (Ronge et al., 1988; Kreuzer et al., 1991). The mRNA abundance of hepatic INSR was highest during the NEB in early lactation and also in cows during the deliberately induced NEB. It appears that the low plasma insulin level causes an upregulation of the INSR, perhaps to maintain the insulin function in the liver, while maximizing nutrient supply to the mammary gland. In dairy cows selected for high milk production, peri- and postparturient insulin resistance plays a pivotal role both in the adaptation to the NEB and in the pathogenesis of some NEB-related diseases, such as excessive lipid accumulation in the liver (Ohtsuka et al., 2001; Grummer, 2008) and ketosis (Hove, 1978). The RQUICKI has been introduced by Holtenius and Holtenius (2007) to detect mild differences in insulin resistance in healthy, lactating dairy cows. Health disorders attributed to the NEB (e.g., ketosis, displacement of the abomasum, or laminitis) were reported to be closely related to the insulin resistance state in dairy cows around parturition (Kerestes et al., 2009). In the study of Kerestes et al. (2009), however, the RQUICKI was not correlated with insulin resistance in dairy cows with ketosis or puerperal metritis. In accordance with Kerestes et al. (2009), our study showed a decrease of the RQUICKI during NEB around parturition, indicating insulin resistance during early lactation and thereby facilitating nutrient uptake by the mammary gland. The RQUICKI remained almost unchanged during the deliberately induced NEB in later lactation (i.e., an insulin resistance did not occur during this period). Stengärde et al. (2010) found the RQUICKI to be a more sensitive method for detection of metabolic imbalances than the individual parameters (NEFA, glucose, and insulin) used for the calculation of the index. As genetically high-yielding dairy cows show a higher insulin resistance than do low-yielding dairy cows (Chagas et al., 2009), the RQUICKI might also be related to differences in productivity.

CONCLUSIONS

Early lactating cows experienced marked changes in the endocrine system and hepatic gene expression in response to the NEB p.p. The deliberately induced NEB at around 100 DIM was unlike early lactation, showing only small alterations of the studied parameters. It was surprising that regulatory mechanisms responded more strongly during the NEB in early lactation when compared with responses during the following deliberately induced NEB by feed restriction, which produced a greater NEB than that of early lactation. Therefore, endocrine and hepatic regulation in dairy cow adaptation to 2 stages of an NEB are different. It seems the

IGFBP, mainly IGFBP-3, are crucial factors to compensate for differences of adaptive changes during NEB in early and midlactation dairy cows. In addition, the development of an insulin resistance to enforce selective nutrient uptake by the mammary gland is most pronounced during NEB in early lactation.

ACKNOWLEDGMENTS

The authors thank Yolande Zbinden and Claudine Morel (Veterinary Physiology, University of Bern, Switzerland) for the blood plasma and gene expression analyses. The mentoring of the Graduate School (Graduate Center Weihenstephan) of the Technical University of Munich (TUM-GS, Freising-Weihenstephan, Germany) during the doctoral study of J. Gross is acknowledged.

REFERENCES

Bauman, D. E., and W. B. Currie. 1980. Partitioning of nutrients during pregnancy and lactation: A review of mechanisms involving homeostasis homeorhesis. J. Dairy Sci. 63:1514–1529.

Bauman, D. E., J. H. Eisemann, and W. B. Currie. 1982. Hormonal effects on partitioning of nutrients for tissue growth: Role of growth hormone and prolactin. Fed. Proc. 41:2538–2544.

Bauman, D. E., and J. M. Elliot. 1983. Control of nutrient partitioning in lactating ruminants. Pages 437–468 in Biochemistry of Lactation. T. B. Mepham, ed. Elsevier Science Publishers, Amsterdam, the Netherlands.

Baxter, R. C. 1993. IGF binding protein-3 and the acid-labile subunit: Formation of the ternary complex in vitro and in vivo. Adv. Exp. Med. Biol. 343:237–244.

Block, S. S., W. R. Butler, R. A. Ehrhardt, A. W. Bell, M. E. Van Amburgh, and Y. R. Boisclair. 2001. Decreased concentration of plasma leptin in periparturient dairy cows is caused by negative energy balance. J. Endocrinol. 171:339–348.

Block, S. S., R. P. Rhoads, D. E. Bauman, R. A. Ehrhardt, M. A. McGuire, B. A. Crooker, J. M. Griinari, T. R. Mackle, W. J. Weber, M. E. Van Amburgh, and Y. R. Boisclair. 2003. Demonstration of a role for insulin in the regulation of leptin in lactating dairy cows. J. Dairy Sci. 86:3508–3515.

Blum, J. W., P. Kunz, H. Leuenberger, K. Gautschi, and M. Keller. 1983. Thyroid hormones, blood plasma metabolites and haematological parameters in relationship to milk yield in dairy cows. Anim. Prod. 36:93–104.

Bradford, B. J., and M. S. Allen. 2008. Negative energy balance increases peripheral ghrelin and growth hormone concentrations in lactating dairy cows. Domest. Anim. Endocrinol. 34:196–203.

Breier, B. H. 1999. Regulation of protein and energy metabolism by the somatotropic axis. Domest. Anim. Endocrinol. 17:209–218.

Butler, S. T., A. L. Marr, S. H. Pelton, R. P. Radcliff, M. C. Lucy, and W. R. Butler. 2003. Insulin restores GH responsiveness during lactation-induced negative energy balance in dairy cattle: Effects on expression of IGF-I and GH receptor 1A. J. Endocrinol. 176:205–217.

Carriquiry, M., W. J. Weber, S. C. Fahrenkrug, and B. A. Crooker. 2009. Hepatic gene expression in multiparous Holstein cows treated with bovine somatotropin and fed n-3 fatty acids in early lactation. J. Dairy Sci. 92:4889–4900.

Chagas, L. M., M. C. Lucy, P. J. Back, D. Blache, J. M. Lee, P. J. S. Gore, A. J. Sheahan, and J. R. Roche. 2009. Insulin resistance in divergent strains of Holstein-Friesian dairy cows offered fresh pasture and increasing amounts of concentrate in early lactation. J. Dairy Sci. 92:216–222.

Chilliard, Y., C. Delavaud, and M. Bonnet. 2005. Leptin expression in ruminants: Nutritional and physiological regulations in relation with energy metabolism. Domest. Anim. Endocrinol. 29:3–22.

Fenwick, M. A., R. Fitzpatrick, D. A. Kenny, M. G. Diskin, J. Patton, J. J. Murphy, and D. C. Wathes. 2008. Interrelationships between negative energy balance (NEB) and IGF regulation in liver of lactating dairy cows. Domest. Anim. Endocrinol. 34:31–44.

Gross, J., H. A. van Dorland, R. M. Bruckmaier, and F. J. Schwarz. 2011. Performance and metabolic profile of dairy cows during a lactational and deliberately induced negative energy balance with subsequent realimentation. J. Dairy Sci. 94:1820–1830.

Grummer, R. R. 2008. Nutritional and management strategies for the prevention of fatty liver in dairy cattle. Vet. J. 176:10–20.

Holtenius, P., and K. Holtenius. 2007. A model to estimate insulin sensitivity in dairy cows. Acta Vet. Scand. 49:29–31.

Hove, K. 1978. Insulin secretion in lactating cows: Responses to glucose infused intravenously in normal, ketonemic, and starved animals. J. Dairy Sci. 61:1407–1413.

Ingvartsen, K. L., and J. B. Andersen. 2000. Integration of metabolism and intake-regulation: A review focusing on periparturient animals. J. Dairy Sci. 83:1573–1597.

Kelley, K. M., Y. Oh, S. E. Gargosky, Z. Gucev, T. Matsumoto, V. Hwa, L. Ng, D. M. Simpson, and R. G. Rosenfeld. 1996. Insulin-like growth factor-binding proteins (IGFBPs) and their regulatory dynamics. Int. J. Biochem. Cell Biol. 28:619–637.

Kerestes, M., V. Faigl, M. Kulcsár, O. Balogh, J. Földi, H. Fébel, Y. Chilliard, and G. Huszenicza. 2009. Periparturient insulin secretion and whole-body insulin responsiveness in dairy cows showing various forms of ketone pattern with or without puerperal metritis. Domest. Anim. Endocrinol. 37:250–261.

Kobayashi, Y., C. K. Boyd, C. J. Bracken, W. R. Lamberson, D. H. Keisler, and M. C. Lucy. 1999. Reduced growth hormone receptor (GHR) messenger RNA in liver of periparturient cattle is caused by a specific down-regulation of GHR 1A that is associated with decreased insulin-like growth factor-I. Endocrinology 140:3947–3954.

Kobayashi, Y., C. K. Boyd, B. L. McCormack, and M. C. Lucy. 2002. Reduced IGF-I after feed restriction in lactating dairy cows is independent of changes in growth hormone receptor 1A. J. Dairy Sci. 85:748–754.

Kreuzer, M., M. Kirchgessner, and J. W. Blum. 1991. Concentrations of hormones and metabolites in blood plasma of cows during and subsequent to different crude protein supply. J. Anim. Physiol. Anim. Nutr. (Berl.) 65:11–20.

Liefers, S. C., R. F. Veerkamp, M. F. W. te Pas, C. Delavaud, Y. Chilliard, and T. van der Lende. 2003. Leptin concentrations in relation to energy balance, milk yield, intake, live weight, and estrus in dairy cows. J. Dairy Sci. 86:799–807.

Lucy, M. C., H. Jiang, and Y. Kobayashi. 2001. Changes in the somatotropic axis associated with the initiation of lactation. J. Dairy Sci. 84(E Suppl.):E113–E119.

McCarthy, S. D., S. T. Butler, J. Patton, M. Daly, D. G. Morris, D. A. Kenny, and S. M. Waters. 2009. Differences in the expression of genes involved in the somatotropic axis in divergent strains of Holstein-Friesian dairy cows during early and mid lactation. J. Dairy Sci. 92:5229–5238.

Meier, S., P. J. S. Gore, C. M. E. Barnett, R. T. Cursons, D. E. Phipps, A. Watkins, and G. A. Verkerk. 2008. Metabolic adaptations associated with irreversible glucose loss are different to those observed during under-nutrition. Domest. Anim. Endocrinol. 34:269–277.

Ohtsuka, H., M. Koiwa, A. Hatsugaya, K. Kudo, F. Hoshi, N. Itoh, H. Yokota, H. Okada, and S. Kawamura. 2001. Relationship between serum tumor necrosis factor-alpha activity and insulin resistance in dairy cows affected with naturally occurring fatty liver. J. Vet. Med. Sci. 63:1021–1025.

Orlowski, C. C., A. L. Brown, G. T. Ooi, Y. W.-H. Yang, L. Y.-H. Tseng, and M. M. Rechler. 1990. Tissue, developmental, and metabolic regulation of messenger ribonucleic acid encoding a rat insulin-like growth factor-binding protein. Endocrinology 126:644–652.

Perseghin, G., A. Caumo, M. Caloni, G. Testolin, and L. Luzi. 2001. Incorporation of the fasting plasma FFA concentration into QUICKI improves its association with insulin sensitivity in non-obese individuals. J. Clin. Endocrinol. Metab. 86:4776–4781.

Pezzi, C., P. A. Accorsi, D. Vigo, N. Govoni, and R. Gaiani. 2003. 5′-Deiodinase activity and circulating thyronines in lactating cows. J. Dairy Sci. 86:152–158.

Radcliff, R. P., B. L. McCormack, D. H. Keisler, B. A. Crooker, and M. C. Lucy. 2006. Partial feed restriction decreases growth hormone receptor 1A mRNA expression in postpartum dairy cows. J. Dairy Sci. 89:611–619.

Renaville, R., M. Hammadi, and D. Portetelle. 2002. Role of somatotropic axis in the mammalian metabolism. Domest. Anim. Endocrinol. 23:351–360.

Ronge, H., J. Blum, C. Clement, F. Jans, H. Leuenberger, and H. Binder. 1988. Somatomedin C in dairy cows related to energy and protein supply and to milk production. Anim. Prod. 47:165–183.

Sauerwein, H., U. Heintges, M. Hennies, T. Selhorst, and A. Daxenberger. 2004. Growth hormone induced alterations of leptin serum concentrations in dairy cows as measured by a novel enzyme immunoassay. Livest. Prod. Sci. 87:189–195.

Stengärde, L., K. Holtenius, M. Tråvén, J. Hultgren, R. Niskanen, and U. Emanuelson. 2010. Blood profiles in dairy cows with displaced abomasum. J. Dairy Sci. 93:4691–4699.

Thissen, J.-P., J.-M. Ketelslegers, and L. E. Underwood. 1994. Nutritional regulation of the insulin-like growth factors. Endocr. Rev. 15:80–101.

van Dorland, H. A., S. Richter, I. Morel, M. G. Doherr, N. Castro, and R. M. Bruckmaier. 2009. Variation in hepatic regulation of metabolism during the dry period and in early lactation in dairy cows. J. Dairy Sci. 92:1924–1940.

Vandehaar, M. J., B. K. Sharma, and R. L. Fogwell. 1995. Effect of dietary energy restriction on the expression of insulin-like growth factor-I in liver and corpus luteum of heifers. J. Dairy Sci. 78:832–841.

Vernon, R. G., R. G. P. Denis, A. Sorensen, and G. Williams. 2002. Leptin and the adaptations of lactation in rodents and ruminants. Horm. Metab. Res. 34:678–685.

Vicari, T., J. J. G. C. van den Borne, W. J. J. Gerrits, Y. Zbinden, and J. W. Blum. 2008. Postprandial blood hormone and metabolite concentrations influenced by feeding frequency and feeding level in veal calves. Domest. Anim. Endocrinol. 34:74–88.

Vicini, J. L., F. C. Buonomo, J. J. Veenhuizen, M. A. Miller, D. R. Clemmons, and R. J. Collier. 1991. Nutrient balance and stage of lactation affect responses of insulin, insulin-like growth factors I and II, and insulin-like growth factor-binding protein 2 to somatotropin administration in dairy cows. J. Nutr. 121:1656–1664.

Windisch, W., M. Kirchgessner, and J. W. Blum. 1991. Hormones and metabolites in blood plasma of lactating dairy cows during and after energy and protein deficiency. J. Anim. Physiol. Anim. Nutr. (Berl.) 65:21–27.

Wook Kim, J., R. P. Rhoads, S. S. Block, T. R. Overton, S. J. Frank, and Y. R. Boisclair. 2004. Dairy cows experience selective reduction of the hepatic growth hormone receptor during the periparturient period. J. Endocrinol. 181:281–290.

Zhao, F. Q., W. M. Moseley, H. A. Tucker, and J. J. Kennelly. 1996. Regulation of glucose transporter gene expression in mammary gland, muscle, and fat of lactating cows by administration of bovine growth hormone and bovine growth hormone-releasing factor. J. Anim. Sci. 74:183–189.

Appendix III

Milk fatty acid profile related to energy balance in dairy cows.

Journal of Dairy Research, Volume 78, pages 479-488, doi:10.1017/S0022029911000550

Gross, J., H.A. van Dorland, R.M. Bruckmaier, and F. J. Schwarz

Milk fatty acid profile related to energy balance in dairy cows

Josef Gross[1], Hendrika A van Dorland[2], Rupert M Bruckmaier[2] and Frieder J Schwarz[1]*

[1] Department of Animal Sciences, Chair of Animal Nutrition, Technical University of Munich, Liesel-Beckmann-Str. 6, D-85350 Freising-Weihenstephan, Germany
[2] Veterinary Physiology, Vetsuisse Faculty, University of Bern, Bremgartenstr. 109a, CH-3001 Bern, Switzerland

Received 2 May 2011; accepted for publication 14 July 2011; first published online 16 August 2011

Milk fatty acid (FA) profile is a dynamic pattern influenced by lactational stage, energy balance and dietary composition. In the first part of this study, effects of the energy balance during the proceeding lactation [weeks 1–21 post partum (pp)] on milk FA profile of 30 dairy cows were evaluated under a constant feeding regimen. In the second part, effects of a negative energy balance (NEB) induced by feed restriction on milk FA profile were studied in 40 multiparous dairy cows (20 feed-restricted and 20 control). Feed restriction (energy balance of −63 MJ NEL/d, restriction of 49% of energy requirements) lasted 3 weeks starting at around 100 days in milk. Milk FA profile changed markedly from week 1 pp up to week 12 pp and remained unchanged thereafter. The proportion of saturated FA (predominantly 10:0, 12:0, 14:0 and 16:0) increased from week 1 pp up to week 12 pp, whereas monounsaturated FA, predominantly the proportion of 18:1,9c decreased as NEB in early lactation became less severe. During the induced NEB, milk FA profile showed a similarly directed pattern as during the NEB in early lactation, although changes were less marked for most FA. Milk FA composition changed rapidly within one week after initiation of feed restriction and tended to adjust to the initial composition despite maintenance of a high NEB. C18:1,9c was increased significantly during the induced NEB indicating mobilization of a considerable amount of adipose tissue. Besides 18:1,9c, changes in saturated FA, monounsaturated FA, de-novo synthesized and preformed FA (sum of FA >C16) reflected energy status in dairy cows and indicated the NEB in early lactation as well as the induced NEB by feed restriction.

Keywords: Milk fat, fatty acids, energy balance, dairy cow.

Milk fat is the main component determining energy expenditure for milk production in dairy cows. It consists almost completely of triglycerides (Moate et al. 2007). Due to proceeding analytical improvements, up to now more than 400 individual fatty acids (FA) in milk fat are documented (Jensen et al. 1991; Moate et al. 2007). During the last decades, milk FA composition has gained the interest of manufacturers and consumers as it influences nutritional, physical and flavour properties of dairy products (Bobe et al. 2007). Changes in the degree of FA unsaturation have an impact on oxidative stability during milk processing (Kay et al. 2005; Glantz et al. 2009). The focus of research regarding the impact of milk FA on human health was especially set on conjugated linoleic acids (CLA) and other polyunsaturated FA (18:2, 18:3) (e.g. Kelsey et al. 2003; Palladino et al. 2009). Dietary manipulation to directly influence the content of these FA is documented in over 100 publications during the last decade (Moate et al. 2007). Thus nutrition is one of the main factors influencing milk FA composition.

Besides diet, lactational stage along with energy balance of dairy cows have an impact on FA profile in cows' milk (Kay et al. 2005; Stoop et al. 2009). During the first couple of weeks after parturition, the occurrence of a negative energy balance (NEB) is common in dairy cows. The deficiency of nutrients and energy is compensated by mobilization of body reserves, predominantly adipose tissue associated with the release of FA. During insufficient supply and quality of feed, a NEB may also occur later in lactation as reported for pastured dairy cows averaging 94 days in milk (DIM) (Leiber et al. 2005). The specific effect of a NEB on milk FA composition was shown in a few earlier studies such as Luick & Smith (1963), who fasted high-yielding dairy cows for 5 d to induce a clinical ketosis or Dann et al. (2005), who enhanced the post partum (pp) NEB by feed restriction.

*For correspondence; e-mail: schwarzf@wzw.tum.de

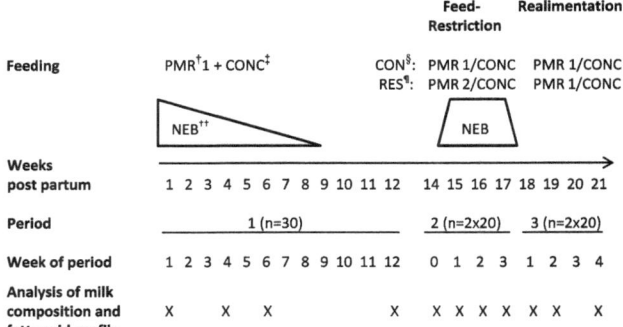

Fig. 1. Experimental design.
† Partial mixed ration
‡ Concentrate
§ Control group
¶ Feed-restricted group
†† Negative energy balance

The focus of the present study is set on the interactions between energy balance and milk FA profile in dairy cows. Contrary to earlier studies, the present study investigated effects of both the NEB in early lactation and a deliberately induced NEB by feed restriction at around 100 DIM.

Materials and Methods

Animal trial

Fig. 1 shows the experimental schedule of the present study. Detailed information on the animal trial and feeding regimen is given in Gross et al. (2011). In brief, the study was conducted with multiparous Holstein dairy cows (3·1 ± 0·2 parities, mean ± SEM) kept in a free stall barn and covered three experimental periods beginning with parturition. Experimental period 1 (from parturition up to week 12 pp) included 40 cows that were treated similarly. However, only milk samples from 30 out of the 40 cows were obtained for FA analysis at all time points in period 1. In period 2 at around 100 DIM (week 14 pp), cows were divided equally into either a control (CON; $n = 20$) or a restriction group (RES; $n = 20$) with feed restriction for 3 weeks (weeks 15 to 17 pp, Fig. 1). After 3 weeks of the deliberately induced NEB, period 3 (weeks 18 to 21 pp, Fig. 1) started, where RES cows were (re)fed similarly to CON cows. Throughout the study, all animals, except RES cows in feed restriction, had free access to a partial mixed ration 1 (PMR 1; 33·7 % grass silage, 44·9 % corn silage, 6·5 % hay and 14·9 % concentrate on a DM basis). Intake of PMR was recorded individually by troughs connected to electronic balances. When milk yield was above 21 kg/d, additional concentrate (CONC, based on barley, wheat, corn kernels, soybean meal, dried sugar beet pulp with molasses) including a vitamin-mineral premix was fed individually according to milk yield in transponder feeding stations (0·4 kg CONC/kg milk; maximum of 8·9 kg CONC/d). In order to induce an energy deficiency of at least 30 % of cows' requirements at the start of period 2, RES cows received a limited amount of a similar diet as the CON cows, but mixed with an additional 25 % of hay (PMR 2) and a limited amount of CONC (0·4 kg/d). Nutrient values of PMR 1, PMR 2 and CONC are described in Gross et al. (2011).

Determination of energy balance

Individual feed intake (PMR and CONC) and milk yield were recorded daily, body weight weekly. Components of the diets were analysed for crude ash, crude fibre, crude protein and crude fat according to the Weende analysis (Naumann et al. 2000) and from that their energy content was calculated according to the German Society of Nutrition Physiology (GfE, 2001). The energy content of PMR 1, PMR 2 and CONC was calculated by multiplying the energy density of the single components with their relative proportion in the diets. Energy content of milk as well as the energetic requirement for maintenance were determined according to GfE (2001). The difference between energy intake by feed and energy expenditure for maintenance and milk production (net energy lactation) results in the energy balance of the individual cow.

Analysis of milk composition, and FA composition of milk and diets

After parturition, cows were milked twice daily (5·00 and 15·00) and milk yield was recorded. Milk samples were pooled once per week from two consecutive milkings, Monday evening and Tuesday morning. Obtained milk aliquots were analysed for milk fat, protein and lactose by an infrared-spectrophotometer (MilkoScan-FT-6000, Foss Analytical A/S, Hillerød, Denmark) in the laboratory of the Milchprüfring Bayern e. V., Wolnzach, Germany. A second aliquot was stored at $-20\,°C$ until analysis for FA composition. Milk FA composition was determined in weeks 1, 4, 6 and 12 pp of period 1, weekly during period 2 and in weeks 1, 2 and 4 of period 3.

Milk fat was extracted according to Bligh & Dyer (1959), modified by Hallermayer (1976). Total fat from feed samples was extracted according to Naumann et al. (2000). FA composition of milk and feed samples was determined using FA methyl esters (FAME) prepared by transesterification with trimethylsulphonium hydroxide (TMSH). FAME were injected into a gas chromatograph (GC 6890, Agilent Technologies, Waldbronn, Germany) with a flame-ionization detector and a DB23 column (Agilent Technologies, Waldbronn, Germany; 60 m × 0·25 mm inner diameter, 0·25 μm film). The carrier gas was hydrogen (constant flow at 1·0 ml/min). Samples were injected by split injection (split ratio 1:100). The oven temperature was increased from 50 °C to 175 °C at 5 deg C per min, from 175 °C to 220 °C at 3·3 deg C per min, held for 7·25 min, increased from 220 °C to 250 °C at 10 deg C per min and held for 5 min. The detector temperature was 260 °C. FA were quantified with Chromeleon 6·8 Chromatography Software (Dionex, Sunnyvale CA, USA) using a FAME mix (Sigma Aldrich, St. Louis MO, USA) as standard. FA composition of PMR 1, PMR 2 and CONC is shown in Table 1.

Statistical analysis

Data presented in text and tables are means ± SEM of individual measurements in each cow. Relations between energy balance and FA were expressed by the Pearson correlation coefficient. Changes in energy balance, feed intake, milk yield, milk composition and milk FA profile over time during lactation and feed restriction with subsequent realimentation were evaluated by a mixed model in SAS, version 9.2 (SAS Institute, Cary NC, USA) with group, week and the group × week interaction as fixed effect. Differences over time and within groups during feed restriction (period 2) and realimentation (period 3) were detected by Bonferroni's t test. P values < 0·05 were considered to be significant.

Table 1. Fatty acid (FA) composition (g/100 g of fatty acid methyl esters, FAME) of experimental diets and concentrate (CONC)

	PMR† 1	PMR 2	CONC‡
Crude fat (g/kg DM)	30	23	21
FA (g/100 g FAME)			
14:0	0·50	0·65	0·19
16:0	16·93	19·97	27·80
16:1,9c	0·28	0·39	0·16
18:0	2·72	2·57	4·18
18:1,9t	0·10	0·12	0·08
18:1,9c	15·90	13·32	20·49
18:1,11c	1·02	0·92	1·47
18:2,9c,12c	37·57	33·36	38·70
18:3,9c,12c,15c	18·59	21·33	2·66
Others and unidentified peaks	6·39	7·38	4·26

† Partial mixed ration
‡ Concentrate

Results and Discussion

Changes in milk composition and milk FA profile with altering energy balance post partum

Data on energy balance, feed intake, milk yield, milk composition and FA profile are shown in Tables 2 and 3. Lactational stage clearly affected daily milk yield and milk composition. Daily milk yield increased up to week 6 pp and declined thereafter (Table 2). Milk fat and protein contents decreased from week 1 pp up to week 6 pp and slightly increased thereafter, whereas lactose content was relatively constant from week 4 pp onwards (Table 2). With progressing lactation and improvement of energy balance through increasing feed intake, especially milk FA profile markedly changed (Table 3). Energy balance in dairy cows was most negative in week 1 pp and improved with increasing feed intake, but was still negative in week 6 pp (Table 2). In order to compensate the insufficient energy intake pp, considerable amounts of body fat are mobilized resulting in elevated plasma concentrations of non-esterified FA (NEFA) and beta-hydroxybutyrate (BHBA). During the NEB in early lactation, plasma glucose concentration in the present study showed a nadir of 3·30 ± 0·04 mmol/l in week 2 pp, whereas plasma concentrations were highest for NEFA in week 2 pp (0·90 ± 0·06 mmol/l) and for BHBA in week 3 pp (0·98 ± 0·14 mmol/l; Gross et al. 2011). After the observed peak of lactation, energy requirements could be met by consumed feed resulting in a positive energy balance.

Basically, milk FA can be derived from four major pathways: the diet, the mammary gland (de-novo synthesis), the rumen (biohydrogenation, bacterial degradation and synthesis), and body fat mobilization (Stoop et al. 2009). Changes in milk FA composition during lactation originate from altered activities in these pathways (Van Knegsel et al. 2005; Stoop et al. 2009).

For the evaluation of changes in milk composition and milk FA profile in the present study with altering energy balance pp depending on the same feeding regimen, data

Table 2. Daily milk yield and milk composition in weeks 1, 4, 6, 12 (all animals), 17 and 21 (control group) post partum. Values without a common superscript letter are significantly different ($P<0.05$)

	Week 1 ($n=30$)	Week 4 ($n=30$)	Week 6 ($n=30$)	Week 12 ($n=30$)	Week 17 ($n=20$)	Week 21 ($n=20$)
Feed intake						
PMR[†] 1, kg DM/d	13.7[b] ±0.3	14.3[b] ±0.3	14.3[b] ±0.3	17.1[a] ±0.4	16.9[a] ±0.4	17.8[a] ±0.5
CONC[‡], kg DM/d	1.6[e] ±0.0	5.7[b] ±0.1	7.6[a] ±0.2	5.8[b] ±0.3	4.7[c] ±0.5	3.6[d] ±0.5
Energy balance						
EB, MJ NEL/d	−45.0[d] ±3.9	−24.8[c] ±3.2	−9.5[b] ±3.1	9.1[a] ±2.7	8.9[a] ±4.7	12.2[a] ±3.1
Milk, kg/d	27.4[c] ±0.8	37.5[a] ±0.8	39.3[a] ±0.9	33.5[b] ±1.2	29.7[c] ±1.3	27.6[c] ±1.2
Fat-corrected milk, kg/d	34.1[b] ±1.2	40.6[a] ±1.1	40.3[a] ±1.1	34.9[b] ±1.2	31.9[bc] ±1.4	29.8[c] ±1.2
Fat, %	5.60[a] ±0.14	4.56[b] ±0.10	4.17[c] ±0.09	4.31[bc] ±0.10	4.48[bc] ±0.08	4.54[b] ±0.09
Protein, %	4.12[a] ±0.06	3.05[d] ±0.04	3.09[d] ±0.04	3.32[c] ±0.05	3.43[bc] ±0.06	3.50[b] ±0.05
Lactose, %	4.46[b] ±0.03	4.77[a] ±0.02	4.79[a] ±0.02	4.76[a] ±0.02	4.75[a] ±0.02	4.72[a] ±0.03

† Partial mixed ration
‡ Concentrate

from all animals in period 1 and CON group in periods 2 and 3 were evaluated in order to investigate the effect of continuous lactation. In the present study, most changes in milk FA profile took place during the observed NEB from weeks 1 to 6 pp, while FA composition was relatively constant between weeks 12 and 21 pp. FA up to 16:0 showed lowest proportions in week 1 pp that increased to relatively constant proportions from week 12 onwards (Table 3). These findings agree with earlier studies (Stull et al. 1966; Palmquist et al. 1993; Kay et al. 2005; Garnsworthy et al. 2006). Confirming results of Stoop et al. (2009), saturated FA (SFA), especially 16:0 increased from weeks 1 to 12 pp in the present study (Fig. 2), while monounsaturated FA (MUFA), mainly represented by 18:1,9c decreased until week 12 pp with improving energy balance (Table 2). The proportion of polyunsaturated FA (PUFA) was relatively constant from week 1 up to week 21 pp (Table 3). Due to the increased adipose tissue mobilization during the NEB in early lactation, preformed FA concentrations (sum of FA >C16) were greatest in week 1 pp and decreased in a similar pattern to that reported by Kay et al. (2005). Oleic acid (18:1,9c) is the predominant FA in adipocytes and primarily released through lipolysis during NEB (Rukkwamsuk et al. 2000). Plasma NEFA and triglycerides are utilized by the mammary gland for milk FA synthesis (Moore & Christie, 1979). The high transfer rate of 18:1,9c from plasma into milk fat (Tyburczy et al. 2008) confirms the elevated proportion of 18:1,9c in milk fat during the NEB pp in the present study. Especially long-chain FA are derived from plasma and incorporated into milk fat (Palmquist et al. 1993) and inhibit the de-novo synthesis of short-chain FA by the mammary gland (Bauman & Davis, 1974). The observed increase in short-chain FA with progressing lactation in the present study is consistent with the decreasing adipose tissue mobilization at around weeks 4–6 pp (Garnsworthy & Huggett, 1992; Palmquist et al. 1993).

Contrary to the findings of Stoop et al. (2009), trans FA slightly increased with improved energy balance of dairy cows in the present study (Table 3). The proportion of CLA in milk fat remained constant from week 1 to week 12 pp and increased slightly thereafter up to week 21 pp. Milk FA from de-novo synthesis ($\leqslant$C14 and part of C16) in the present study increased from week 1 pp up to week 12 pp (Fig. 2) in agreement with Palmquist et al. (1993) and Kay et al. (2005). Although the FA synthesized de novo comprise approximately 40% by weight over the entire lactation, preformed FA contribute a larger portion of the total FA in early lactation (Kay et al. 2005). Percentage of preformed FA decreased up to week 12 pp in the present study. Thereafter milk composition and milk FA profile were stable until the end of the study. Garnsworthy et al. (2006) concluded that stage of lactation does not affect the relative incorporation of de-novo synthesized and preformed FA when the composition of diets remains constant. Because of the same feeding regimen in the present study, changes in milk FA profile regarding de-novo synthesized and preformed FA therefore reflect changes in energy balance of dairy cows.

Changes in milk and milk FA composition during feed restriction and subsequent realimentation

Due to feed restriction in period 2, RES cows experienced a significant NEB in weeks 15 to 17 pp being even more intense compared with the NEB occurring in the first 6 weeks

Table 3. Milk fatty acid (FA) composition (g/100 g of fatty acid methyl esters, FAME) in weeks 1, 4, 6, 12 (all animals), 17 and 21 (control group) post partum. Values without a common superscript letter are significantly different ($P<0.05$)

FA (g/100 FAME)	Week 1 (n=30)	Week 4 (n=30)	Week 6 (n=30)	Week 12 (n=30)	Week 17 (n=20)	Week 21 (n=20)
4:0	3·85^a ±0·12	3·54^b ±0·11	3·38^b ±0·08	3·14^c ±0·07	3·10^c ±0·07	3·15^c ±0·07
6:0	2·21^c ±0·11	2·41^{ab} ±0·08	2·55^a ±0·05	2·40^{abc} ±0·06	2·39^{abc} ±0·04	2·34^{bc} ±0·04
8:0	1·16^c ±0·08	1·39^b ±0·06	1·58^a ±0·04	1·50^{ab} ±0·04	1·51^{ab} ±0·03	1·49^{ab} ±0·02
10:0	2·24^c ±0·18	2·82^b ±0·16	3·52^a ±0·13	3·52^a ±0·10	3·61^a ±0·08	3·56^a ±0·06
10:1	0·12^d ±0·01	0·21^c ±0·01	0·27^b ±0·01	0·31^{ab} ±0·01	0·32^a ±0·01	0·34^a ±0·01
12:0	2·37^c ±0·20	2·96^b ±0·18	3·83^a ±0·18	4·07^a ±0·13	4·27^a ±0·11	4·26^a ±0·08
12:1	0·03^e ±0·00	0·05^d ±0·00	0·07^c ±0·01	0·09^b ±0·00	0·10^{ab} ±0·00	0·10^a ±0·00
14:0iso	0·07^b ±0·00	0·06^b ±0·01	0·07^b ±0·01	0·08^b ±0·01	0·10^a ±0·00	0·11^a ±0·01
14:0	8·82^c ±0·48	9·75^b ±0·32	11·36^a ±0·28	12·06^a ±0·23	12·18^a ±0·17	12·22^a ±0·14
14:1,9c	0·62^b ±0·04	1·58^a ±0·04	1·00^a ±0·08	1·17^a ±0·12	1·07^a ±0·05	1·36^a ±0·13
15:0	0·64^c ±0·03	0·74^c ±0·05	0·98^b ±0·09	1·15^{ab} ±0·07	1·22^a ±0·04	1·17^a ±0·04
16:0iso	0·18^c ±0·01	0·17^c ±0·01	0·17^c ±0·01	0·20^{bc} ±0·01	0·22^{ab} ±0·01	0·24^a ±0·01
16:0	28·77^c ±0·61	29·62^c ±0·63	31·38^b ±0·64	35·62^a ±0·70	36·75^a ±0·49	36·23^a ±0·39
16:1,9c	2·31^a ±0·16	2·27^a ±0·14	1·93^b ±0·12	1·84^b ±0·08	1·78^b ±0·06	1·82^b ±0·05
17:0	0·46^a ±0·01	0·38^b ±0·02	0·37^b ±0·02	0·38^b ±0·02	0·36^b ±0·01	0·34^b ±0·01
17:1,9c	0·37^a ±0·02	0·35^a ±0·02	0·26^b ±0·02	0·22^{bc} ±0·02	0·19^c ±0·01	0·19^c ±0·01
18:0	12·88^a ±0·33	10·87^b ±0·29	10·17^b ±0·36	8·92^c ±0·28	8·56^c ±0·22	8·54^c ±0·17
18:1,9t	0·40 ±0·03	0·39 ±0·02	0·42 ±0·01	0·42 ±0·01	0·40 ±0·01	0·42 ±0·01
18:1,11t	1·01^{bc} ±0·09	0·94^c ±0·05	1·06^{bc} ±0·04	1·11^{ab} ±0·05	1·15^{ab} ±0·04	1·23^a ±0·04
18:1,9c	25·75^a ±1·22	23·96^a ±1·05	19·89^b ±0·89	16·16^c ±0·69	15·00^c ±0·46	15·30^c ±0·24
18:1,11c	1·06^a ±0·09	1·01^{ab} ±0·09	0·92^{abc} ±0·07	0·76^{bcd} ±0·08	0·68^{cd} ±0·06	0·63^d ±0·05
18:1,12c	0·24^c ±0·01	0·25^c ±0·01	0·26^{bc} ±0·01	0·26^{bc} ±0·01	0·29^{ab} ±0·01	0·29^a ±0·01
18:2,9c,12c	1·95 ±0·05	1·89 ±0·06	1·94 ±0·06	1·84 ±0·05	1·79 ±0·04	1·77 ±0·04
18:3,9c,12c,15c	0·38^{ab} ±0·01	0·34^{bc} ±0·01	0·35^{bc} ±0·01	0·33^c ±0·01	0·40^a ±0·01	0·39^a ±0·01
18:2,9c,11t	0·35^b ±0·02	0·34^b ±0·02	0·34^b ±0·01	0·37^b ±0·01	0·43^a ±0·01	0·48^a ±0·02
18:2,10t,12c	0·04 ±0·01	0·03 ±0·01	0·03 ±0·01	0·02 ±0·01	0·03 ±0·01	0·03 ±0·01

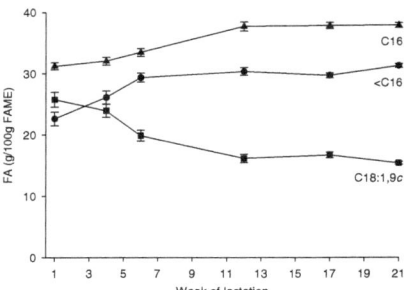

Fig. 2. Proportions (g/100 g of fatty acid methyl esters, FAME) of de-novo synthesized FA (<C16; circles), C16 FA (triangles) and C18:1,9c (squares) in milk fat during the first 21 weeks of lactation in dairy cows.

of lactation (Tables 2 and 4). Besides energy supply the dietary composition also was changed in the group of RES cows during period 2 as the amount of the PMR and the concentrate was limited. Additionally, PMR 2 fed to RES cows included more hay than the PMR 1 fed to CON cows. Despite the higher induced NEB by feed restriction compared with the NEB in early lactation, plasma NEFA and BHBA concentrations were elevated only moderately in RES cows compared with CON cows during period 2 (0·23±0·02 v. 0·14±0·01 mmol/l and 0·62±0·03 v. 0·52±0·02 mmol/l, respectively).

Milk fat content was elevated during feed restriction for RES cows (Table 4). Changes in milk yield and composition have been discussed in Gross et al. (2011). Data on the effect of energy balance on milk fat composition are scarce (Stoop et al. 2009). In the present study, milk FA profile of CON cows was stable during the whole time of periods 2 and 3. For RES cows, the proportion of most FA ≤ 16:0 (e.g. 6:0, 10:0, 10:1, 12:0, 14:0, 16:0) was decreased during the NEB induced by feed restriction compared with the respective initial values, whereas preformed FA, especially 17:1,9c, 18:0 and 18:1,9c arising from body fat mobilization increased markedly during feed restriction (Table 5). These changes occurred rapidly within the first week of feed restriction (on average 3 d distance between the start of feed restriction and the next milking sample) and disappeared completely within one week of realimentation (4 d on average). The proportion of CLA in milk fat of RES cows was elevated at the start of feed restriction and adjusted immediately to initial values (Table 5). The rise of CLA in RES cows may be attributed to the changed diet towards less concentrate and more roughage. Despite the maintenance of the deliberately induced NEB by feed restriction at a relatively constant level, FA showed a tendency during the NEB to adjust towards the initial levels with progressing feed restriction. The pattern of decreasing short-chain FA and increase of long-chain FA during an induced NEB was reported in an earlier study of Luick & Smith (1963). During feed restriction (period 2), SFA decreased, while MUFA (especially 18:1,9c) increased for RES cows compared with CON cows (Fig. 3). PUFA were stable during period 2 and the following realimentation period in RES cows (Table 5).

Luick & Smith (1963) examined whether changes in milk FA composition during feed restriction are caused by a decreased synthesis of short-chain FA or by an increased incorporation of long-chain FA absorbed from plasma. According to Luick & Smith (1963), the failure to utilize beta-hydroxybutyrate occurs when its concentration in plasma is elevated, i.e. during fasting and ketosis. This in turn, accounts for the relatively high levels of oleic acid found in milk fat of fasting and ketotic cows (Luick & Smith, 1963) as observed in the present study. Although less in their extent, milk FA in the present study clearly showed a similar pattern during a deliberately induced NEB by feed restriction at around 100 DIM compared with the NEB in early lactation. Compared with milk of dairy cows in positive energy balance (week 14 pp), proportions for single FA (e.g. 17:1,9c; 18:1,9c) were changed up to 80% during the NEB in early lactation and during the deliberately induced NEB by feed restriction.

Van Haelst et al. (2008) determined whether concentrations of specific FA in milk fat are suitable for the early detection of subclinical ketosis as mobilization of adipose tissue precedes development of ketosis (Reist et al. 2003). Van Haelst et al. (2008) suggested the elevated proportion of 18:1,9c as an interesting trait for prediction of subclinical ketosis, particularly since this FA was elevated in milk fat before diagnosis of ketosis. As milk FA changed with altering energy balance, it is obvious to identify milk FA indicating a NEB in dairy cows independent of their lactational stage. Therefore, correlations between milk FA and the energy balance of all cows were calculated. Correlation over all cows between energy balance and the proportion of 18:1,9c was 0·77. We wanted to investigate whether the correlation is higher in cows with a higher NEB. Thus the correlation between energy balance and the proportion of 18:1,9c in milk fat of 5 cows with the most negative EB in week 1 pp (−80·2 MJ NEL/d) was calculated, but did not show a closer relationship (r=0·62). The correlation between EB and 18:1,9c for RES cows with the highest NEB in the first week of feed restriction (−83·2 MJ NEL/d) was 0·92. From these results, an elevated proportion of 18:1,9c in milk fat can be confirmed to be a suitable marker for a NEB. The correlation between energy balance and a single FA during the NEB in early lactation and during the deliberately induced NEB ranged from 0·71 to 0·96. However, the low proportion and relatively high variation in changed FA (e.g. 11:0; 12:1; Tables 3 and 5) restrict the predictive value of these FA to indicate a NEB although changes were significant between RES and CON cows. On the contrary, the correlation between energy balance and groups of FA was higher in cows with a more intense NEB during feed

Table 4. Milk yield and milk composition for feed-restricted (RES) and control cows (CON) during feed restriction and realimentation. For differences over time within group, values without a common superscript are significantly different ($P>0.05$), significant differences between RES- and CON-group within week are marked with * ($P<0.05$)

	Restricted Group ($n=20$)								Control Group ($n=20$)							
	Period 2				Period 3			Period 2				Period 3			
Week	0	1	2	3	1	2	0	1	2	3	1	2				
Feed intake																
PMR†, kg DM/d	17·0ᵃ ±0·7	9·4ᵃᶜ ±0·3	9·6ᵃᶜ ±0·3	9·8ᶜ ±0·3	15·6ᵃᵇ ±0·4	16·9ᵃ ±0·5	16·4ᵃᵇ ±0·5	15·6ᵇ ±0·3	17·3ᵃ ±0·5	16·9ᵃ ±0·4	16·3ᵃᵇ ±0·4	17·0ᵃ ±0·5				
CONC‡, kg DM/d	5·5ᵃ ±0·5	1·2ᵃᵈ ±0·1	0·4ᵃᵉ ±0·0	0·4ᵃᵉ ±0·0	2·9ᵃᶜ ±0·3	4·2ᵇ ±0·4	5·4 ±0·5	5·2 ±0·5	4·8 ±0·5	4·7 ±0·5	4·4 ±0·4	4·3 ±0·5				
Energy status																
EB§, MJ NEL/d	9·9ᵃ ±2·8	−68·0ᵃᶜ ±2·8	−64·7ᵃᶜ ±3·9	−61·8ᵃᶜ ±4·2	−4·6ᵃᵇ ±2·7	6·2ᵃ ±3·3	3·7 ±2·9	0·8 ±3·2	8·1 ±3·8	8·9 ±4·7	5·8 ±3·5	9·9 ±3·6				
Milk, kg/d	33·4ᵃ ±1·2	29·3ᵇᶜ ±1·1	27·9ᵇ ±1·0	27·2ᶜ ±0·9	28·3ᵇᶜ ±1·1	30·4ᵃᵇ ±1·3	32·3 ±1·5	31·1 ±1·4	31·1 ±1·3	29·7 ±1·3	28·8 ±1·1	28·8 ±1·3				
FCM¶, kg/d	33·6ᵃ ±1·0	31·8ᵃ ±1·1	29·0*ᵇᶜ ±0·9	28·6*ᶜ ±0·9	28·9ᵇᶜ ±1·1	31·3ᵃᵇ ±1·1	34·2ᵃ ±1·2	32·8ᵃᵇ ±1·4	33·0*ᵃᵇ ±1·2	31·9*ᵃᵇ ±1·4	30·8ᵃᵇ ±1·1	30·6ᵇ ±1·2				
Fat, %	4·11*ᵃᵇ ±0·13	4·64ᵃ ±0·17	4·31ᵃᵇ ±0·12	4·38ᵃᵇ ±0·14	4·19ᵇ ±0·13	4·28ᵃᵇ ±0·15	4·50 ±0·19	4·41 ±0·11	4·45 ±0·11	4·48 ±0·08	4·49 ±0·13	4·48 ±0·13				
Protein, %	3·38ᵃᵇ ±0·06	3·21*ᵇᶜ ±0·06	3·18*ᵃᶜ ±0·06	3·18*ᵃᶜ ±0·07	3·33ᵃᵇᶜ ±0·05	3·43ᵃ ±0·05	3·41 ±0·06	3·41 ±0·05	3·41 ±0·05	3·43 ±0·06	3·43 ±0·06	3·48 ±0·06				
Lactose, %	4·80ᵃ ±0·02	4·79ᵃ ±0·02	4·80ᵃ ±0·02	4·75ᵃᵇ ±0·02	4·71ᵇ ±0·02	4·73ᵇ ±0·03	4·74 ±0·04	4·77 ±0·03	4·76 ±0·03	4·75 ±0·02	4·74 ±0·03	4·73 ±0·03				

† Partial mixed ration
‡ Concentrate
§ Energy balance
¶ Fat-corrected milk

Table 5. Milk fatty acid (FA) composition (g/100 g fatty acid methyl esters, FAME) for feed-restricted (RES) and control cows (CON) during feed restriction and realimentation. For differences over time within group, values without a common superscript are significantly different ($P>0.05$), significant differences between RES- and CON-group within week are marked with * ($P<0.05$)

	Restricted Group (n=20)												Control Group (n=20)											
	Period 2				Period 3									Period 2			Period 3		
Week	0	1	2	3	1	2	0	1	2	3	1	2
FA (g/100g FAME)												
4:0	2.97 ±0.07	3.03 ±0.10	3.15 ±0.11	3.17 ±0.12	3.21 ±0.13	3.13 ±0.11	3.08 ±0.08	3.10 ±0.05	3.17 ±0.12	3.10 ±0.07	3.10 ±0.07	3.03 ±0.05
6:0	2.35^a ±0.06	2.15^{ab} ±0.04	2.30^{ab} ±0.06	2.32^{ab} ±0.07	2.45^a ±0.08	2.42^a ±0.03	2.41 ±0.04	2.38 ±0.04	2.46 ±0.06	2.40 ±0.05	2.41 ±0.05	2.34 ±0.03
8:0	1.51^a ±0.04	1.29^b ±0.03	1.36^{ab} ±0.03	1.38^{ab} ±0.04	1.53^a ±0.04	1.54^a ±0.04	1.53 ±0.03	1.49 ±0.04	1.55 ±0.03	1.51 ±0.04	1.52 ±0.03	1.47 ±0.03
10:0	3.60^a ±0.08	2.79^{ab} ±0.10	2.96^{ab} ±0.09	3.05^{ab} ±0.10	3.59^a ±0.10	3.64^a ±0.10	3.73 ±0.09	3.54 ±0.11	3.70 ±0.09	3.61 ±0.11	3.62 ±0.10	3.48 ±0.08
10:1	0.36^a ±0.01	0.27^c ±0.01	0.29^{abc} ±0.01	0.32^b ±0.01	0.39^{aa} ±0.01	0.38^{aa} ±0.01	0.34 ±0.01	0.32 ±0.01	0.33 ±0.01	0.32 ±0.01	0.33 ±0.02	0.32 ±0.01
12:0	4.27^a ±0.08	3.18^b ±0.13	3.32^b ±0.13	3.49^{ab} ±0.13	4.34^a ±0.13	4.37^a ±0.13	4.47 ±0.13	4.16 ±0.15	4.35 ±0.12	4.27 ±0.14	4.28 ±0.13	4.10 ±0.10
12:1	0.11^b ±0.00	0.07^{cd} ±0.00	0.08^{acd} ±0.00	0.09^c ±0.01	0.13^{aa} ±0.01	0.12^{aa} ±0.00	0.10 ±0.00	0.09 ±0.01	0.10 ±0.00	0.10 ±0.00	0.10 ±0.01	0.10 ±0.00
14:0iso	0.08^b ±0.01	0.09^{ab} ±0.01	0.10^a ±0.01	0.10^{ab} ±0.00	0.08^{ab} ±0.01	0.09^b ±0.01	0.09 ±0.00	0.09 ±0.01	0.09 ±0.00	0.10 ±0.00	0.11 ±0.01	0.10 ±0.01
14:0	12.38^a ±0.16	10.95^{ab} ±0.29	11.38^{ab} ±0.22	11.46^b ±0.22	12.26^a ±0.21	12.29^a ±0.18	12.36 ±0.19	12.00 ±0.28	12.20 ±0.22	12.18 ±0.24	12.29 ±0.22	12.03 ±0.25
14:1,9c	1.40^{ab} ±0.13	1.14^b ±0.10	1.21^{ab} ±0.10	1.27^{ab} ±0.08	1.50^a ±0.12	1.50^a ±0.14	1.13 ±0.05	1.07 ±0.06	1.08 ±0.05	1.07 ±0.05	1.14 ±0.06	1.51 ±0.12
15:0	1.44^a ±0.09	1.00^{ab} ±0.05	1.01^{ab} ±0.05	1.04^b ±0.04	1.26^a ±0.06	1.37^a ±0.09	1.29 ±0.07	1.21 ±0.07	1.26 ±0.09	1.22 ±0.07	1.24 ±0.07	1.22 ±0.07
16:0iso	0.18^b ±0.01	0.24^a ±0.01	0.24^a ±0.01	0.22^{ab} ±0.01	0.20^b ±0.01	0.19^{ab} ±0.01	0.21 ±0.01	0.21 ±0.01	0.22 ±0.01	0.22 ±0.02	0.22 ±0.01	0.23 ±0.02
16:0	36.14^{ab} ±0.61	32.63^{cd} ±0.67	33.51^{cd} ±0.69	34.58^{abc} ±0.74	37.84^a ±0.62	36.03^{ab} ±0.51	37.35 ±0.64	36.52 ±0.75	36.38 ±0.73	36.75 ±0.55	36.43 ±0.69	36.52 ±0.78
16:1,9c	1.86 ±0.08	1.94 ±0.09	1.91 ±0.08	1.93 ±0.08	2.06 ±0.09	1.95 ±0.08	1.85 ±0.08	1.86 ±0.11	1.80 ±0.08	1.78 ±0.08	1.84 ±0.08	1.83 ±0.10
17:0	0.39 ±0.02	0.39 ±0.01	0.37 ±0.02	0.36 ±0.02	0.34 ±0.02	0.36 ±0.02	0.37 ±0.01	0.37 ±0.01	0.36 ±0.01	0.36 ±0.01	0.36 ±0.01	0.36 ±0.01
17:1,9c	0.21^b ±0.01	0.28^{aa} ±0.02	0.26^{aa} ±0.01	0.25^{aa} ±0.01	0.21^b ±0.01	0.21^b ±0.01	0.20 ±0.01	0.21 ±0.01	0.19 ±0.01	0.19 ±0.01	0.20 ±0.01	0.19 ±0.01
18:0	8.22^b ±0.19	10.09^{aa} ±0.22	9.86^{aa} ±0.29	9.46^{aa} ±0.35	7.44^{*b} ±0.32	8.19^b ±0.25	8.02 ±0.25	8.56 ±0.41	8.51 ±0.33	8.56 ±0.24	8.53 ±0.36	8.49 ±0.39

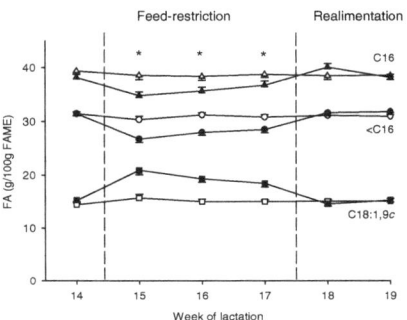

Fig. 3. Proportions (g/100 g of fatty acid methyl esters, FAME) of de-novo synthesized FA (<C16; circles), C16 FA (triangles) and C18:1,9c (squares) in milk fat of feed-restricted cows (filled symbols) and control cows (empty symbols) during feed restriction (weeks 15–17 post partum) and subsequent realimentation (weeks 18–19 post partum). Stars indicate a significant difference between the groups ($P < 0.05$).

restriction that ranged from 0·92 up to 0·98 for SFA, MUFA (predominantly 18:1,9c), de-novo synthesized (sum of FA<C16, $r = 0.94$) and preformed FA (sum of FA >C16, $r = 0.92$). The higher proportion of these summarized FA in milk fat makes their changes a more appropriate tool reflecting energy balance in dairy cows compared with a single FA represented at a low concentration.

Conclusions

Post-partum changes in milk FA profile in the present study followed previous findings. Short- and medium-chain FA up to C16 increased with the decreasing NEB pp, while long-chain FA, especially 18:1,9c decreased as mobilization of body fat reserves declined. The responses of FA profiles of cows' milk due to a NEB at two lactational stages in the present study – the NEB in early lactation and the deliberately induced NEB by feed restriction – was similarly directed. Despite the maintenance of a high NEB during the feed restriction period, changes in milk FA profile were less pronounced compared with changes during the NEB in early lactation and tended to adjust to the initial composition. However, milk FA profile changed within a few days after initiation of the deliberately induced NEB and showed no more differences within the first week of realimentation compared with control cows. For the dietary composition and feeding regimen in the present study, the close relationship with energy balance makes changes in 18:1,9c as well as in groups of FA (SFA, MUFA, de-novo synthesized and preformed FA) suitable indicators of the energy balance in dairy cows.

References

Bauman DE & Davis CL 1974 Biosynthesis of milk fat. In: *Lactation—A comprehensive treatise Vol. 2* (Eds BL Larson & VR Smith) p. 31. New York, USA: Academic Press

Bligh EG & Dyer WJ 1959 A rapid method of total lipid extraction and purification. *Canadian Journal of Biochemistry and Physiology* **37** 911–917

Bobe G, Lindberg GL, Freeman AE & Beitz DC 2007 Short communication: Composition of milk protein and milk fatty acids is stable for cows differing in genetic merit for milk production. *Journal of Dairy Science* **90** 3955–3960

Dann HM, Morin DE, Bollero GA, Murphy MR & Drackley JK 2005 Prepartum intake, postpartum induction of ketosis, and periparturient disorders affect the metabolic status of dairy cows. *Journal of Dairy Science* **88** 3249–3264

Garnsworthy PC & Huggett CD 1992 The influence of the fat concentration of the diet on the response by dairy cows to body condition at calving. *Animal Production* **54** 7–13

Garnsworthy PC, Masson LL, Lock AL & Mottram TT 2006 Variation of milk citrate with stage of lactation and de novo fatty acid synthesis in dairy cows. *Journal of Dairy Science* **89** 1604–1612

GfE (German Society of Nutrition Physiology) 2001 [Recommendations on energy and nutrient requirements of dairy cows and rearing cattle], ed. Ausschuss für Bedarfsnormen der Gesellschaft für Ernährungsphysiologie. DLG-Verlag, Frankfurt am Main, Germany

Glantz M, Lindmark Mansson H, Stalhammar H, Barström L-O, Fröjelin M, Knutsson A, Teluk C & Paulsson M 2009 Effects of animal selection on milk composition and processability. *Journal of Dairy Science* **92** 4589–4603

Gross J, van Dorland HA, Bruckmaier RM & Schwarz FJ 2011 Performance and metabolic profile of dairy cows during a lactational and deliberately induced negative energy balance with subsequent realimentation. *Journal of Dairy Science* **94** 1820–1830

Hallermayer R 1976 [A rapid method to determine fat content in food]. *Deutsche Lebensmittelrundschau* **10** 356–359

Jensen RG, Ferris AM & Lammi-Keefe CJ 1991 The composition of milk fat. *Journal of Dairy Science* **74** 3228–3243

Kay JK, Weber WJ, Moore CE, Bauman DE, Hansen LB, Chester-Jones H, Crooker BA & Baumgard LH 2005 Effects of week of lactation and genetic selection for milk yield on milk fatty acid composition in Holstein cows. *Journal of Dairy Science* **88** 3886–3893

Kelsey JA, Corl BA, Collier RJ & Bauman DE 2003 The effect of breed, parity, and stage of lactation on conjugated linoleic acid (CLA) in milk fat from dairy cows. *Journal of Dairy Science* **86** 2588–2597

Leiber F, Kreuzer M, Nigg D, Wettstein H-R & Scheeder MRL 2005 A study on the causes for the elevated n-3 fatty acids in cows' milk of alpine origin. *Lipids* **40** 191–202

Luick JR & Smith LM 1963 Fatty acid synthesis during fasting and bovine ketosis. *Journal of Dairy Science* **46** 1251–1255

Moate PJ, Chalupa W, Boston RC & Lean IJ 2007 Milk fatty acids. I. Variation in the concentration of individual fatty acids in bovine milk. *Journal of Dairy Science* **90** 4730–4739

Moore JH & Christie WW 1979 Lipid metabolism in the mammary gland of ruminant animals. *Progress in Lipid Research* **17** 347–395

Naumann K, Bassler R, Seibold R & Barth C 2000 [The chemical analysis of feedstuffs. Book of methods no. III], ed. Verband Deutscher Landwirtschaftlicher Untersuchungs- und Forschungsanstalten. Darmstadt, Germany: VDLUFA-Press

Palladino RA, O`Donovan M, Murphy JJ, McEvoy M, Callan J, Boland TM & Kenny DA 2009 Fatty acid intake and milk fatty acid composition of Holstein dairy cows under different grazing strategies: Herbage mass and daily herbage allowance. *Journal of Dairy Science* **92** 5212–5223

Palmquist DL, Beaulieu AD & Barbano DM 1993 ADSA foundation symposium: Milk fat synthesis and modification. Feed and animal factors influencing milk fat composition. *Journal of Dairy Science* **76** 1753–1771

Reist M, Erdin D, von Euw D, Tschuemperlin K, Leuenberger H, Delavaud C, Chilliard Y, Hammon HM, Kuenzi N & Blum JW 2003 Concentrate feeding strategy in lactating dairy cow: Metabolic and endocrine changes with emphasis on leptin. *Journal of Dairy Science* **86** 1690–1706

Rukkwamsuk T, Geelen MJH, Kruip TAM & Wensing T 2000 Interrelation of fatty acid composition in adipose tissue, serum, and liver of dairy cows during the development of fatty liver postpartum. *Journal of Dairy Science* **83** 52–59

Stoop WM, Bovenhuis H, Heck JML & van Arendonk JAM 2009 Effect of lactation stage and energy status on milk fat composition of Holstein-Friesian cows. *Journal of Dairy Science* **92** 1469–1478

Stull JW, Brown WH, Valdez C & Tucker H 1966 Fatty acid composition of milk. III. Variation with stage of lactation. *Journal of Dairy Science* **49** 1401–1405

Tyburczy C, Lock AL, Dwyer DA, Destaillats F, Mouloungui Z, Candy L & Bauman DE 2008 Uptake and utilization of trans octadecenoic acids in lactating cows. *Journal of Dairy Science* **91** 3850–3861

Van Haelst YNT, Beeckman A, van Knegsel ATM & Fievez V 2008 Short communication: Elevated concentrations of oleic acid and long-chain fatty acids in milk fat of multiparous subclinical ketotic cows. *Journal of Dairy Science* **91** 4683–4686

Van Knegsel ATM, van den Brand H, Dijkstra J, Tamminga S & Kemp B 2005 Effect of dietary energy source on energy balance, production, metabolic disorders and reproduction in lactating dairy cattle. Review. *Reproduction Nutrition Development* **45** 665–688

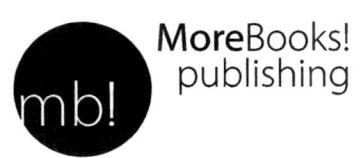
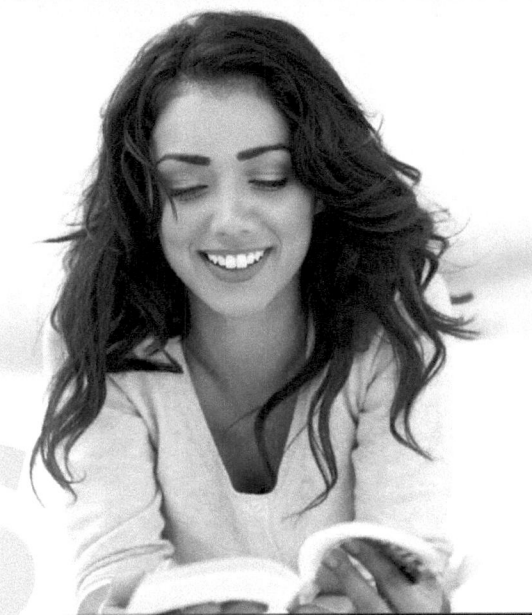

i want morebooks!

Buy your books fast and straightforward online - at one of world's fastest growing online book stores! Environmentally sound due to Print-on-Demand technologies.

Buy your books online at
www.get-morebooks.com

Kaufen Sie Ihre Bücher schnell und unkompliziert online – auf einer der am schnellsten wachsenden Buchhandelsplattformen weltweit! Dank Print-On-Demand umwelt- und ressourcenschonend produziert.

Bücher schneller online kaufen
www.morebooks.de

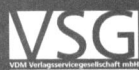

VDM Verlagsservicegesellschaft mbH
Heinrich-Böcking-Str. 6-8
D - 66121 Saarbrücken

Telefon: +49 681 3720 174
Telefax: +49 681 3720 1749

info@vdm-vsg.de
www.vdm-vsg.de

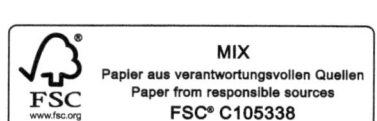

Printed by Books on Demand GmbH, Norderstedt / Germany